Based on research at the famous City Gym, sponsored by the Sports Council, the exercises in this book are designed to get you fit in a matter of weeks.

Two or three *short* sessions a week, in your home, without equipment, can give you a new-found sense of vigour and liveliness and help keep you from joining the 200,000 who die prematurely each year from heart attacks.

D1512849

Malcolm Carruthers and Alistair Murray

# F/40 Fitness on 40 Minutes a Week

Futura Publications Limited

A Futura Book

First published in Great Britain in 1976
by Futura Publications Limited

ISBN: 0 8600 7324 6
Printed in Great Britain by
Hazell Watson & Viney Ltd
Aylesbury, Bucks

Futura Publications Limited
Warner Road,
London SE5

# FOREWORD
## by Sir Roger Bannister

Most people are unfit and alarmingly content to be so; perhaps because our Great British Character refuses to be bullied by those intent on doing us good. Too many of us slump with flabby limbs and tired minds watching television and let middle age spread all over us. There are, of course, many paths to fitness through sport and recreation; exercises are not to everyone's taste but this remarkable book could give everyone a second chance. Diligent readers will be far less likely to join the 200,000, who, each year, die prematurely of heart attacks — a national tragedy that we could do so much to avoid. Any reservations you may have about starting on the road to positive health will melt away, cajoled by Dr. Malcolm Carruther's sound medical knowledge and lucid prose. Any embarrassment you may feel will be dispelled by Al Murray's lifelong success at inspiring people with his own enthusiasm. Among the hidden benefits may well be the realization for example that cigarette smoking and exercise are incompatible. After only a matter of weeks with this good book at your side you should be delightedly surprised at a new-found health and vigour, and the habit could become life-long.

I am delighted to recommend this book.

# FOREWORD
by Sir Robin E. Brook, CMG, CBE

It is gratifying to me, as Chairman of the Sports Council, that one of our research studies should result in a book such as this one which, I am sure, will help people of all ages both to enjoy and to benefit from a programme of exercises.

This is a 'no-nonsense' book. The authors, each in his own way so experienced in recommending and supervising exercise as a means of keeping fit or overcoming the effects on the body of sedentary work, write simply and directly yet always with a respect for the reader's intelligence.

*Fitness for All*, certainly; but as this book originated from a study of exercise and the middle-aged man, it is my earnest hope that people in this age group in particular will pay great attention to it. Malcolm Carruthers and Al Murray *do* know what they are talking about.

# AUTHORS' ACKNOWLEDGEMENTS

Our thanks are due, firstly, to the many people who helped in the development, testing and application of methods of physical training in unfit adults.

At the City Gym, Margaret Holfeld and Frank Shipman have given unfailing help in the training of members and charting their progress. Throughout, Dr. Janet Carruthers has carried out a great deal of the work involved in the collection and collation of the material for this book. The typescript of this and the related articles were prepared by Miss Patten-Thomas.

The formal study of the medical benefits of this type of exercise was pioneered in this country by the late Dr. Harold Lewis of the Medical Research Council, and continued under the guidance of Dr. Otto Edholm.

Dr. Peter Nixon, Cardiologist to the Charing Cross Hospital in London was instrumental in applying gymnasium treatment to patients with a wide variety of cardiovascular disorders, and in monitoring the effects of this form of cardiac rehabilitation.

Drs. Richard Edwards, Neil Pride, Marie Hutchinson and Steven Spiro of the Hammersmith Hospital helped in the physiological assessment of its effects, and Dr. Cecily de Moncheaux studied its psychological aspects.

Financial support for the study was provided by the Sports Council, Medical Research Council and the British Heart Foundation.

# CONTENTS

# INTRODUCTION

'I keep six honest serving-men
(They taught me all I knew);
Their names are what and why and when,
And how and where and who'.

Here, although not in order, are some answers to Rudyard
Kipling's six questions applied to exercise. Many people, feeling instinctively restless and ill at ease in their physically inert
city lives, think about taking up exercise. Too often instead
they take the advice to lie down until the feeling wears off.
There are several reasons for this. Firstly, most of us are 'also
rans' in competitive sports and are afraid of looking silly if, in
middle-age or later, we are seen exercising. Secondly, we are
showered with widely differing advice on exercise by the radio,
television, newspapers and magazines, most of which is ill-
informed, untested, and even occasionally downright dangerous. Thirdly, few people realize the wide range of benefits
of carefully controlled progressive exercise, while the few
dramatic cases of harm arising from over-exertion, usually due
to ignoring the principles of exercising in safety and comfort,
receive wide publicity. It is to show the benefits and make
exercise safe for all by reference to the lessons learned in studying the physical training of unfit people in the Sports Council
sponsored study at the City Gym, that this handbook is produced.

It also gives a scheme of mobility exercises, followed by a
schedule of training with light weights, for people who would
like to exercise in the privacy of their own homes.

# CHAPTER ONE

# WHY
*Why bother to exercise?*

The biggest obstacle to exercising is inertia. Sloth comes naturally to us all, and is undeniably as popular today as when it was first listed as one of the seven deadly sins over one thousand years ago. It is only relatively recently, however, that thanks to city living, modern transport and labour saving devices, large numbers of people have been able to savour the delights of sloth.

Delightful at first and in small doses, it then becomes a habit and later a disease that is difficult to shake off. In middle-age it is likely to be self-perpetuating because of stiffness, fatness and perhaps even shortness of breath from heart or lung trouble.

There are several good reasons, therefore, why to get the most out of your life, both in quantity and quality, you need enough exercise to keep fit. Not super-fit, bulging biceps fit, minute-miler fit, rugger-scrum fit, or jolly hockey-sticks fit. Just plain medium fit, because as was recognized as long ago as Greek and Roman times, an active mind needs to be balanced by an active body. Let's go through some of the benefits of being fit:

*Feel better:* Your ancestors who came down from the trees a mere one or two million years ago weren't basically different from you in brain power, emotions or body chemistry. Your space-age life and surroundings are, however, vastly different. You don't have to walk or run many miles each day to get food. You don't have to shiver in damp cold caves to keep warm in winter. You've mostly got convenience foods and comfortable homes with labour saving gadgets and a car at the door. That's fine – that's progress – that's civilization. What does it cost?

Firstly, you have to rely much more on brain power than

muscle power. Secondly, living in cities is a crowded, noisy, competitive business, and to survive you have to join the rat race. Thirdly, people, places, ideas and values are changing rapidly, producing a condition which has aptly been called 'culture shock'.

However, this combination does make life interesting, exciting and challenging. It is one of the reasons why people flock to the cities, which they find stimulating but occasionally stressful. City life seems to turn them on. Turning on is probably a chemical process. Mankind has a mass of automatic biochemical responses to various types of emotion. Research recently carried out with the British Heart Foundation helped us to show that positive emotions such as anger, aggression, frustration and competition, gave the body a shot of a powerful hormone called noradrenaline. Negative emotions, such as anxiety or uncertainty, whether brought on by free-fall parachuting or the sight of a dentist's drill, were found to produce the closely related but better known hormone adrenaline.

Large amounts of the noradrenaline hormone were found to be in the blood of racing drivers and athletes tested after their very different types of race. It could be regarded as being the 'kick hormone' which prepares both mind and body to 'get up and go'. The motor trade would say it puts a tiger in your tank. Many experiments suggest that it can make you more alert, reduce tiredness, help concentration, and act as a general stimulant. Because of its pleasant effects on the mind, it can be a self-administered drug of addiction. People find by experience various ways of turning on the body's supplies.

Some can produce it by an almost conscious effort of will. Some get it by putting themselves in exciting situations, jet-set travel, or by living in a gay social whirl. Others find, like James Bond, that smoking, sex, sadism, or just getting passionately involved in anything, is sufficient to produce the effect. Now probably the safest way of producing it is by exercise. This way you get the mental stimulation but prevent the undesirable side effects of the drug by using up the fat which it releases into the blood stream. At the same time, exercise prevents most of the rise in blood pressure which would otherwise be caused, by diverting blood to the dilated vessels in the active muscles. Thus the reactions of body and mind are balanced in a natural and healthy way, so that both greatly benefit.

*Enjoy better health*

As far as long-term fitness goes, there is no doubt that being overweight and having flabby muscles contribute to osteo-arthritis, back pain, breathing problems and even make you accident prone. It is harder for you to dodge the bus or the bus to dodge you if you're two or three stone overweight. One of the jobs muscles have to do is to act as springs to strengthen, stabilize and cushion joints, particularly in the spine. Any car owner knows that if his springs are flat, the suspension is soon ruined. This may be why one definition of modern man is a constipated biped with a bad back.

There is also a lot of evidence to suggest that if you take just a moderate amount of vigorous exercise of the type described later in this book, your chances of developing one of the big killers of our time, heart attacks and high blood pressure, are very much reduced. This was demonstrated, for example, last year in a study which compared mildly energetic civil servants defined as those taking over half an hour of any of a wide range of vigorous activities during the week, with inert ones who didn't. The number of heart attacks in the energetic was about a third of those in the inert. The activity does seem to need to be relatively brisk to get definite benefit however, as studies of other groups walking various short distances to work showed little or no protective effect. Workers in occupations which involve heavy manual labour are, however, recognized as being relatively immune to heart attacks when compared with those in sedentary jobs.

Why exercise should have this protective effect is not known. Some people put it down to physical reasons such as lowering weight, blood pressure and blood fat levels. Others think that it also acts on emotional factors, lessening stress and tension. Either way its advantages in promoting positive health are being increasingly recognized by the medical profession.

There are even financial benefits to being fit. If you can get your weight and blood pressure down by exercise, your new life insurance premiums are likely to be less. This has been carried to the stage in Germany where some companies offer special low rates to people willing to exercise regularly in recognized gymnasia offering special facilities. Both insurers and the insured appear to benefit greatly!

*Sleep better:* Exercise relaxes you, lessens the tensions of everyday life, and helps you get a good night's sleep. This is a matter of common experience, and is constantly found in physical training courses of all types. Again, the reason is unknown, but the effect tends to be most marked in really unfit and anxious people. Though difficult to measure, the majority of people notice that previously disturbed sleep patterns are restored to normal within a few weeks of beginning progressive training in the gymnasium.

*Eat better:* While not suggesting that you should eat more, exercise improves your appetite, so that you get greater enjoyment from what you eat. As you begin to feel the other benefits of getting fitter, you may come to limit the amount you eat so as to avoid getting that overfull, lethargic feeling which is experienced particularly after a large mid-day meal. At the same time, if you like your food, as most people do, you can stay on quite a generous diet when exercising and yet not gain weight.

Discouraging comparisons are often made between energy used up in exercise and energy taken in when you eat or drink. Typical of these is the saying that you have to walk a mile to work off one glass of sherry. Fortunately, this probably isn't a fair comparison as there is some recent evidence that once you get your muscles into training again the enzymes in them will continue to use up energy at a faster rate even when you are not actually exercising. Heat loss from a thin person is also greater than from a fat one, so these are two ways in which the exerciser can lose weight even while sitting still.

*Look better:* Last but not least, looking better reinforces the fact that you feel better. Although you probably won't become Mr. Universe or Miss World, a better build, a flatter stomach and loss of a few inches round the waist is likely to improve the way in which yourself and others see you. Keep it up, and you'll probably find several of your fat and flabby friends will join you as they can't stand the social competition.

# CHAPTER TWO

# WHAT

*What happens when you exercise?*

A lot is known about people at the two extremes of fitness, the very fit 5% of the population and the sick 5%. The middle 90%, the fit and unfit, have largely been ignored.

The very fit, including competitive sportsmen and spacemen have been intensively studied, both to make them able to excel still further and because there is a fascination in exploring the limits of human endurance and performance. This top physical rank of mortals have been measured in every possible way and in every conceivable situation. Their glorious bodies have been filmed in action, measured, weighed and even examined under microscopes. Their performance is constantly rated and assessed in terms of strength, speed, skill and endurance, as well as by the amount of success they have in their particular field of endeavour.

On the medical side, these superb specimens and a few fit young medical students have again been examined in action. Those who study 'how the various functions of the body are performed', the physiologists, began by measuring work load, oxygen consumption, energy expenditure, the electrical activity in muscles, and circulatory changes. Biochemists then added their observations on the chemical changes in the muscles and blood during exercise, so that a large amount of very detailed information was gathered.

Perhaps not surprisingly, they found the same changes occur in the body during exercise as in any animal preparing for an emergency in which it will have to fight or run away. The emergency control centre in the mid-brain responds by organizing a 'red-alert' throughout the body. To do this, it has overriding control within the so-called 'autonomic nervous system'. This system is made up of nerves which run from the brain to all parts of the body, automatically and largely subconsciously regulating and co-ordinating their activity according to the needs of the moment. Being automatic and practically instantaneous, it had great survival value for our ancestors, as they did not have to sit and think for half an hour of ways of tuning up the body to prepare for running away from a tiger. One look and you're off, the body fully adapted to get up and go.

It is worth looking a bit more closely at this autonomic nervous system to find out how it prepares the body for both physical and mental activity. It has two parts with generally opposing actions, the so-called sympathetic and parasympathetic divisions. The sympathetic side is concerned with preparing the body for states of war, and the parasympathetic with times of peace. As the activity of one waxes, so the other usually wanes, otherwise they would largely cancel each other out.

There are many similarities between a country preparing for war and the action of the sympathetic getting the body ready for 'fight or flight'. To start with, messages are sent by telegraph and telephone (nerves) and via the other media (hormones) announcing the emergency and saying what needs to be done to meet it. These are the main stress hormones, noradrenaline and the better-known adrenaline. Noradrenaline, produced in greater amounts in 'fight' situations, has the immediate effect of making you mentally more alert as described in Chapter 1. It also turns on your oil supplies in the form of free active fat from the body's fat stores, and increases the amount going to those parts of the body which need it, in two ways. Firstly, it opens up blood vessels going to the muscles, and shuts down those going to the gut. Secondly, it increases the rate of flow by pushing up the blood pressure.

Adrenaline, produced in greater amounts in 'flight' situations, mobilizes another form of fuel, glucose, and speeds this on its way to the muscles by putting up heart rate. It also makes it easier for the body to burn these fuel supplies, increasing the supply of oxygen by widening the air passages in the lungs, and arranges for cooling as you run away by increasing sweat rates. This explains some of the changes which are obvious in anxious or frightened people.

The parasympathetic system, being more peaceable, is concerned with building up fuel supplies. It does this by increasing traffic (blood flow) to and from the ports (stomach and intestines) and chemically helping the accumulation of stores of fat and sugar. It also slows down the heart and narrows the air passages, putting a brake on most activities. If you want to see the parasympathetic working, look at a person asleep after a large meal.

All this leads up to an explanation of what happens during exercise. At rest there is a low level of activity in the sympathetic system balanced by a low level in the parasympathetic. As a first move, when exercise begins gradually, parasympathetic activity ceases. With little or no additional sympathetic activity, its now unopposed action causes the heart to speed up to over 100 beats per minute and increases the flow of blood together with the fat, sugar and oxygen which it contains, to the muscles. In more intensive exercise, these changes are insufficient to meet the needs of the vigorously contracting muscles, and so the sympathetic drive increases with heart rate, rising to a maximum in top-line athletes around 200 beats per minute, and all the other changes described becoming fully effective.

One very important practical point arising from this theoretical discussion of changes in the balance of sympathetic and parasympathetic activity during exercise is the setting of the upper and lower limits of intensity of effort which is appropriate to various degrees of fitness. Interestingly enough, two very different lines of study have given similar answers. The research on unfit middle-aged business executives on which this book is based, suggested that the pulse rate during the exercise period had to be raised to over a 100 beats per minute for any useful training effect to occur. Above this level the benefit increases steadily with pulse rate until a maximum rate consistent with comfort and safety is reached. Similarly, the study of the leisure activities of civil servants suggested that only occupations which might be regarded as sufficiently vigorous to raise the pulse rate to above 100 exerted a dramatic effect in reducing the heart attack rate.

These studies both seem to indicate that lowering parasympathetic activity on its own is not enough, but that you need to increase sympathetic activity with exercise to gain much physical benefit. The period during which you are building up the size, strength, blood supply and activity of your muscles, and burning up surplus fat and sugar in the process, is not limited just to the time you are exercising. These benefits of a single exercise session carry on for several days or even weeks, which is encouraging to those who don't want to exercise daily, but only two or three times a week.

Just as there is a lower limit of intensity below which the value of exercise falls off sharply, so there is an upper limit beyond which no additional advantage is gained, and a lot may be lost by over-exertion. On a pulse basis, this upper limit even in entirely healthy individuals falls steadily with age, as described in Chapter 5. Warning that you have reached this point is usually in the form of severe breathlessness, muscle cramps or general distress. While athletes can drive themselves through this pain barrier to levels of physical achievement not even approached by the majority of people, there is no point in it during non-competitive fitness training. Considerable danger arises when unfit, or even moderately fit people push themselves to or through this upper limit. It doesn't have to hurt to do you good!

# CHAPTER THREE

# WHO
*Who needs exercise? Who is going to instruct?*

Exercise, most people agree, would do everybody good. Everybody except themselves that is. So who does really need it?

Few would actively recommend exercise for a baby for instance. It exercises what little muscle it has throughout its waking hours by waving its arms and legs in the air, sucking in food and forcing it out, and crying loudly on every possible occasion. During this stage its parents get the exercise they need by carrying it round, pushing a pram and washing the nappies.

Infants exercise themselves without any kind of instruction, unless forcibly confined. For their size, they are so active that one adult Olympic athlete who tried to imitate every movement that a free-range five year old made in a day, ended up completely exhausted. Infancy is an important period of muscle and bone development and they really need full scope for this intensive activity, which shapes their bodies and physical skills, like balance and co-ordination, for a lifetime. Habits of activity or inactivity, of posture and of over-eating, are often established before the child starts formal education at the age of five. Restrictions at this stage, such as being confined to a flat because the mother can't leave the toddler in a playground several floors below, and has to resort to pacifying it with television and sweets, can produce a fat, lethargic child which grows to become a fat lethargic adult.

During school years, there is generally plenty of physical activity, although games are generally competitive and, apart from the few who are able to excel, many become discouraged and leave school as spectators rather than participants. There has, however, in recent years been an encouraging growth in activities such as gymnastics and swimming, where large numbers of people can join in and reach their own enjoyable level of proficiency. This trend has been encouraged by schemes such as the graded awards of the British Amateur Gymnastics Association and the Amateur Swimming Association.

Those in their twenties and thirties usually get enough physical activity with mating, home-building and child rearing. Also some continue their school sports such as football, tennis or squash. These are less than ideal forms of exercise because, as described later, they are erratic in intensity and competitive in nature. Also, as the men who play them progress in their business, trade or profession, such play tends to be overtaken by work and household commitments. One expression of this progressive fall-off in participation in exercise is the large number of overweight people in their thirties seen at medical examinations for life insurance. Heart attacks are also becoming far more common in this age group.

Women are relatively immune from heart disease until they are over forty. Most housewives will tell you that they get plenty of exercise anyway looking after young children, keeping the home clean and shopping.

It is the middle-aged unfit male in his forties and fifties for whom exercise has the most to offer. Yet this is the very person most reluctant to take it up. Middle-age spread has often caught up with him, which discourages exertion and may make him loth to appear in shorts or a bathing suit. He may also be deeply immersed in his work and not like to compete, or even exercise alongside, the younger and obviously fitter men at his office or factory, for fear of unfavourable comparisons being made.

This is understandable but sad, as it is just when diseases of the heart and circulation take their biggest toll, and together with degenerative joint conditions and breathlessness, prevent a man enjoying fully his family life and fruits of his earlier labours. It is also largely unnecessary, because a small amount of regular but vigorous exercise would prevent many of these conditions developing.

Women in their forties and fifties would also often benefit from exercise as the lessening of the physical work of looking after children often leads to weight and joint trouble or high blood pressure. Even so, heart trouble remains far less of a problem than with their husbands as, up to the age of fifty-five women only get one-sixth of the number of heart attacks suffered by men.

Those in their sixties and seventies are often mistakenly thought to be past exercising, and are laughed at if they try. Those, however, who have taken up exercise with due caution even at a late age, or better still have kept it up throughout adult life, often live on fit and well, have the last laugh on younger detractors of exercise. Several very tough and happy senior citizens, including Sir Laurence Olivier and Victor Sylvester, bear eloquent testimony to this at the City Gymnasium.

'You're as young as your arteries' is a good motto at all ages, but especially in the elderly. It is then that the same degenerative changes called atheroma begin seriously to affect the arteries in the brain, as they do at an earlier age in the heart. Although there is not a great deal of medical evidence for it, it appears that the physically active also remain mentally active for longer, and certainly enjoy life far more. Also movement prevents joints from stiffening up and keeps the bones strong, so that there are many fringe benefits to exercise at all ages.

*Who is going to instruct?*

One point on which adult physical educationists will agree is that there are not enough of them to go round. This applies to whether they are physical training instructors, remedial gymnasts or physiotherapists by training. Because of this shortage, the considerable overlap of their fields of endeavour, and the presence of unsuspected abnormalities in the people they instruct, there appears to be little need for demarcation disputes, and a lot to learn from each other.

In schools, for example, supervision of the full range of exercise may be the responsibility of a games master who sometimes has had formal training in the principles and practice of the diverse activities and sometimes not. Even many of the best school instructors do not tell the pupils the reasons why exercise for all can lay the foundation for a lifetime of health, but just tell them to get on and do it this way or that. Such positive health education is unfortunately rare at the time when it could do a great deal of good.

Young adults are increasingly well cared for in this country as far as recreational facilities go, as many sports facilities are designed with them in mind, and there is little need for caution as their bodies can stand any reasonable strain. However, the unfit middle-aged and elderly are relatively poorly treated, as they are often shy about sharing the same facilities as younger, stronger people, and if they do so they either drive themselves or are driven to over-exertion. There is a great lack of physical educationists with specific training in the problems and needs of unfit adults taking up exercise. This needs to take into account the fact that up to a third of adult males taking up exercise in middle-age may have undiagnosed diseases of the heart and circulation, as well as the extreme caution and careful progressive mobilization needed to prevent joint disorders.

We would like to suggest that there is enormous potential for improving the health of the nation if the need for and uses of exercise are explained at an early age, and that pleasant, and above all safe forms of exercise can be provided for at every age.

# CHAPTER FOUR

# WHEN
*When should you exercise? When should you not?*

The National Press and the Media in general are on what might be described as a 'fitness kick' at present. This particularly applies to diet, which produces a spring fever of activity in the form of newspaper and magazine articles when people survey the disastrous effects that a winter's over-eating and under-exercising has on their figures. People are also waking up to the fact that even if a physical activity doesn't guarantee longevity, it certainly improves the quality of your life. In spite of this glut of advice and encouragement and the many health and fitness clubs which have sprung up all over the country in the last 10 years, the question of when to exercise, and perhaps more importantly, when not to, are hardly if ever raised. Thousands must have been discouraged, and some even damaged their health because of lack of appreciation of the importance of the 'when' question.

The American craze for jogging is a good example. Soon after it was introduced, it became popular right across the country as a sort of cult, like hoola-hooping or streaking, something that could be talked about at parties. Like these other activities, it was assumed that everyone who felt like it could do it, and that supervision or instruction was superfluous. Many of the unfittest and fattest American men dashed out into the streets and countryside, and jogged up and down enthusiastically. Little attention was paid to timing, style or the weather. Participation was what mattered, and often a competitive element of keeping up with, or preferably overtaking, Mr. Jones crept in. Some benefited greatly for the short time they took this form of exercise, whilst others got backache, strained muscles and sprained joints. A few even dropped dead in their tracks in their track-suits. As bad news is good news to newspaper men, the wide publicity which these unfortunate episodes received in both the lay and medical press spread a cloud of suspicion over exercise in general, and that form of it in particular. For lack of a few elementary precautions, the popularity of the pastime declined rapidly.

Experience in helping very unfit people and heart patients to start exercising again, often after they have been doing little except sitting and lying since they left school, has aided the development of some important ideas on when is the best and safest time. Although a lot more research is needed in this field, we think the same general principles apply to any type of exercise for adults and so it is worth taking a detailed look at this list of 'when' factors.

*When do you need to exercise?*
When you wake up stiff every morning and find that your everyday activities are limited by difficulty in bending, turning and twisting.
When you find that any extra physical effort, such as carrying something heavy or running for a bus, either can't be managed or leaves you a panting, unhappy wreck for some minutes afterwards.
When you can't walk briskly along on the flat and talk at the same time if you feel like doing so.
When you can no longer find the time to play your favourite game, which may demand more time travelling than playing.
When a normal day's work leaves you physically exhausted and you find yourself taking much longer than usual to recover from fatigue.
When you regularly can't get to sleep because of over-tiredness and tension and you still feel tired the next day.
When your usual mood becomes one of pessimism or depression.
When you look at your naked shape in the mirror and don't like what you see.
When the bathroom scales protest as well.
When you feel like it.

Having decided you need to exercise, the next move is to decide on when you will really be ready to do so. Some prepara-

27

tions may be needed. Firstly, is there any medical reason why you shouldn't start yet? If you are in any doubt, play safe and consult your doctor. Symptoms which need checking include pain in the chest or arms, or severe shortness of breath on exertion, and back or joint troubles.

Are you a heavy smoker? This beyond any reasonable doubt, is one of the most damaging habits you can have from the health point of view. Luckily, a fringe benefit of exercises is that it can help you to stop smoking, as most people soon find out how periods of heavy smoking reduce their fitness as measured by their ability to do these schedules. Also most people get tired of this form of personal pollution, and when they feel more relaxed with increasing fitness, find it easier to give up. If you are a smoker, however, you should start the vigorous part of this exercise programme with extra caution, as it can make you from 10 to 20 years older than your real age in exercise terms, as well as in looks!

How much overweight are you? Your weight should drop steadily towards normal when you start exercising, unless you allow your appetite to run riot at the same time. If you are severely overweight, say by more than three stone above the so-called ideal weight for a person of your sex and height, for safety's sake begin by dieting. There are probably books, pamphlets, articles and diet sheets weighing about two to three stone for every overweight person in the country. If all this material was put together into one compendium of diet, you wouldn't need to read it. Just picking it up and putting it down twenty times a day would be enough!

More seriously though, there are many good books on the subject of how to reduce your weight, and if you really follow the advice in any of them for a month or two, unless you have one of the rare biochemical disorders causing diet-resistant obesity, your weight will come down to a reasonable level where you can exercise with safety and comfort. One of the best and cheapest of such books is by the nutrition expert, Professor John Yudkin, and is called 'This Slimming Business'. His basic suggestion is that if you cut most of the sugar and starch out of your diet you can, within reason, eat pretty well whatever else you like in the way of protein and fats, and forget about calorie counting and the other drearier rituals of slimming.

Having decided that at least if you are not fit you are not ill either, the next step is to define your objectives. Just how fit do you want to be, and in what particular way? These are questions the novice exerciser seldom asks himself and even if he does, often he can't obtain the advice required to answer them unless he intends to take up a particular sport under the guidance of a proficient coach. He may read many articles on the subject of fitness and yet end up more confused than he started, as they are usually written by people with little or no practical experience of the special problems of physical training of unfit adults.

The two commonly used terms 'Health' and 'Fitness' are often confused. At its lowest level, health could be described as the absence of disease, even though nearly all the efforts of the National Health Service is directed to the treatment of disease. Taken a stage further, health is also a state of mind – what the French describe as 'joie de vivre'. Only when we have got this combination of physical and mental well-being can we consider ourselves healthy.

Fitness is another matter, as it can be defined in terms of a person's ability to reach a particular level of physical activity. The basic ingredients of a training course for a man who wants to take up some sporting activity in his spare time, one who wants to improve his physique or even the heart patient undergoing rehabilitation therapy, usually differ not so much in type as the points on the intensity scale at which they start and then finally level off.

Having thought of the general degree of fitness you want and think you can reasonably attain, you can then decide on your order of priority among the three S's of suppleness (mobility), strength and stamina (endurance). Although we will be describing exercises to bring about all three of these aims, you may wish to emphasize one of them. Even so, especially if you are starting at a low level of fitness, you are advised always to begin with the simple mobility exercises given at the beginning of the next chapter to prepare you for the strength and endurance exercises which follow.

At the same time as you are starting the mobility exercises, not feeling ready for the other more strenuous forms of exertion, you may wish to work up to them gradually by other forms of light exercise, such as walking or cycling. Taking the same safety precautions as described for the gymnasium exercise, you can progress in easy stages by increasing the distance and pace at which you walk, for example. Learning to walk before you can run is not just a proverb: It's the basis of exercising safely.

Having planned your programme, get cracking – or should we say creaking. When is the best time of day? Perhaps in loving memory of the ritual early morning physical training sessions in the army, many people imagine that the crack of dawn, when the frost is still on the ground, has some special virtue. If it is so, our research hasn't been able to show it. Apart from the fact that your spouse may be laughing at you from under the bedclothes as you leap round the house or garden in the light of the rising sun, there are several good scientific reasons why mid-morning, before lunch or the early evening are probably preferable times.

Firstly, however alert your mind may be, the body definitely takes time to reach its peak of performance. While you are waking up, activating hormones such as noradrenaline and cortisol are tuning up the nerves and muscles, and pumping fat and sugar into the blood stream to give you the energy to get up and go. Most people find that it takes most of their available strength to fight their way through the morning rush hour to work, and feel lethargic and disinclined to do anything much until they have had their morning coffee. Joints also tend to be stiff first thing in the morning, and the body needs to be warm to exercise in comfort. Further, cold pushes up the blood pressure as we demonstrated in people leaping into the icy-cold waters of Hampstead and Highgate swimming ponds at Christmas. It may be very invigorating when you are used to it, but to the unacclimatized it seems a rather unnecessary test of the strength of the heart and lungs.

Neither is after a heavy business lunch the best time of day for exercise. Apart from any difficulty you may have in bending, so much blood is diverted to the stomach and intestines to cope with the inrush of food, that there is little to spare for the muscles, and you may get muscle cramps if nothing worse.

Lastly, don't leave it too late in the day when you are mentally exhausted and your body is wanting to sign off for the night and has to be pushed into activity.

From these considerations on when to exercise, the times when it is important not to do so becomes obvious:

When you already feel over-tired
When you have even a minor illness like a cold or 'flu
When it's too cold
When your rhythm of exercise slows down, and the movements become too laboured
When your recommended exercise pulse rate is being exceeded
and above all, when you have to push yourself to go on.

# CHAPTER FIVE

# HOW
## *How do you begin? How do you progress?*

Having taken the advice on when to exercise you are now presumably ready and eager to begin, and want to know how much should be done in the early stages. Many people in the first flush of enthusiasm often start at too high a work load considered in terms of exercise 'volume' and intensity. This is at best unnecessary and painful in terms of strained muscles and joints, and at worst may throw a sudden strain on the heart. Ego makes us attempt too much, combined with the fact that you may feel all right at the time, but it catches up with you later. Begin as if you were an unfit old lady! It's easier and safer to speed up when you are surer of your level of fitness.

Even in the schedule we have laid down, you can begin with less than our minimal repetitions. Caution is encouraged, as you may not be able to tell how these exercises affect you until the next day. So play it cool, and you will be thrilled to find most days that not only can you do a little more each session, but also that any starting problems you get are limited to a very mild stiffness in the muscles, which can be a pleasant reminder that you have really made a start.

Another factor which can deceive you is the strength of your muscles, which is often greater than the efficiency of the heart and lungs. This causes you to start off briskly enough and yet, in a short time, your heart is thumping and you may be puffing and panting. It is one of the reasons why pulse control has been found at the City Gym to be so useful in the safe regulation of exercise. There, the same principle is applied, but under careful supervision and with an age 'handicap' of not less than 20 years, to people starting rehabilitation two or three months after a heart attack. Drugs which artificially slow the heart, such as the increasingly prescribed $\beta$-blocking compounds used in treating high blood pressure and other circulatory disorders, undo this safety-belt. Those with heart trouble or high blood pressure should consult their doctors on this point. If in doubt, find out!

Learning to take your pulse rate is simple. Assuming you are wearing a watch on your left wrist, take the tips of the fingers of the left hand and place them on the inside of the right wrist quite near the base of the thumb of the right hand. You will then find the pulse very easily. Count the beats for six seconds on your watch, multiply by ten and that's the rate per minute. The maximum safe pulse levels are shown on the chart for people of different ages and degrees of fitness. The importance of keeping to the pulse ranges shown on this chart cannot be over-emphasized. The appropriate rate must not be exceeded. It's like the need to change up smoothly through the gears when driving a car; start in top gear and you may stall the engine, perhaps permanently.

You may, in the early days, find you have to rest between exercises to keep the pulse rate down. Later, when the level of training of your heart and lungs improves, you will be able to reduce and eventually eliminate the rest pauses. As your fitness increases, you will find that you are able to do a great deal more work for a relatively lower pulse rate. Pulse control also enables you to work at a lower pulse rate when you are a little more tired than usual, as well as giving some feedback information on the effect of adverse influences such as smoking, over-eating and over-work, on the condition of your body. This, together with not getting to the point where you strain yourself to keep going, is the essential guide to exercising in safety.

The schedules in this book are in no way designed to produce champion athletes or sportsmen. Their objectives may be summarized by the word SAFE, which stands for Safe, Acceptable, Fitness-producing and Economic. Safety is built into the course by the type of exercise and gradual build-up under pulse control. Acceptability is essential, as the best exercise system on earth is useless unless it is used on a regular basis. This is produced by having a varied series of exercises and making them easy and convenient to carry out. Fitness in the sense of a feeling of well-being, or improved strength and mobility, is the

33

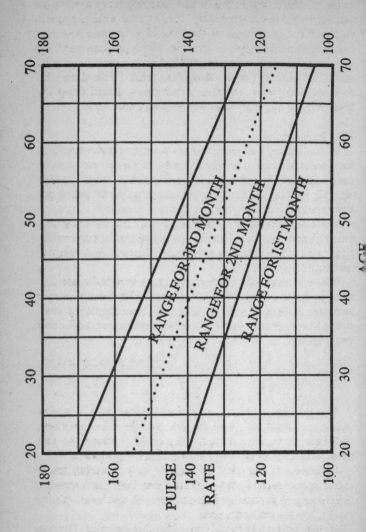

aim of most who take up exercise. Economy is provided in terms of time by the fact that these exercises only need to be carried out for two or preferably three 15 to 20 minute sessions each week. Our research at the City Gym showed how this 'condensed recipe' type of exercise could produce very big benefits for a small outlay in terms of time, space and equipment. Not only did people taking this minimal dose of exercise look and feel better, but their blood pressure and blood fat levels fell in a medically most encouraging way.

## How to begin

Having chosen a suitable time of day, you should exercise in loose warm clothing if the room is cold. If you are very unfit or overweight go through a token performance of stage one cutting the starting times or repetitions by half, and resting between each exercise until you get fitter.

The stages described are based on a combination of mobility, strength and endurance exercises, and are gently progressive. Start with stage one and work steadily through, following the instructions.

When you are ready to progress to stage two, and eventually to stage three still include the stage one mobility routine. Stages two and three are built on what you have already accomplished, and you will notice how these exercises are made more progressive;

| Strength exercise (arms) 1 | Table press-ups Stage 1 |
| ,,   ,,   ,, 2 | Chair   ,,   ,, 2 |
| ,,   ,,   ,, 3 | Floor   ,,   ,, 3 |

The principle involved in the strength exercises is to first provide minimal resistance for the muscles being exercised, and then progress by changing the starting position so that more weight has to be moved by the exercising muscles.

Endurance is improved principally by performing movements against much lighter resistance than in strength training, progressing by an increase in the number of repetitions or time rather than the resistance used.

You are now ready to start your Mobility exercises. Perform them at a moderate speed, without haste or jerkiness.

35

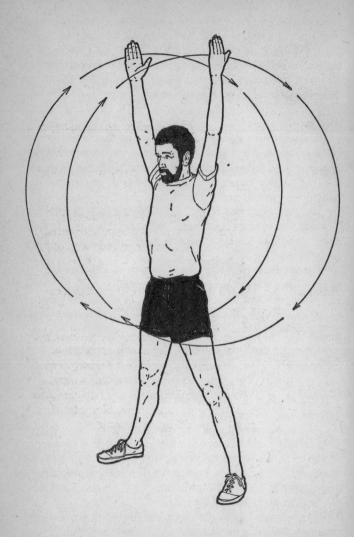

| | |
|---|---|
| Exercise 1 | Arm circling |
| Purpose | To mobilize the shoulder and chest region and to improve posture |
| Start | Feet very wide apart, trunk erect, arms by sides |
| Movement | Raise both arms forwards, upwards to overhead, then lower sideways to starting position. Perform in a quiet continuous movement |
| Breathing | In on the upward movement, out as you return to starting position |
| Repetitions | This also applies to the following exercises in this section. Begin with 10 complete movements. A complete movement ends when you return to the starting position. Progress over the next few weeks of regular exercise to 15 or 20 times. Aim to brush your ears with the upper arms |

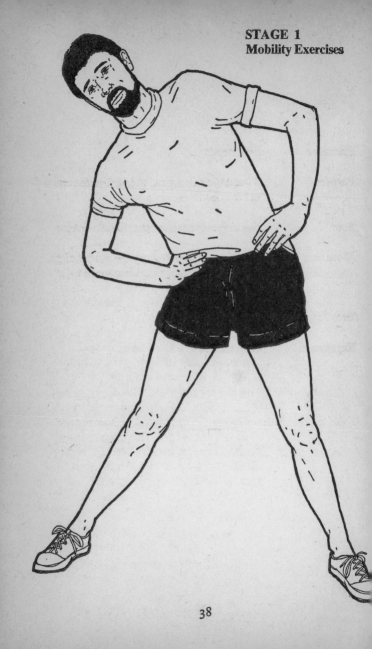

| | |
|---|---|
| Exercise 2 | Side bends |
| Purpose | To mobilize the spine, to improve the range of side bending |
| Start | Stand feet very wide apart, hands on hips |
| Movement | Bend first to the left, keep the head at right angles to the trunk, then bend to the right without jerking |
| Breathing | Freely throughout |
| Repetitions | As Exercise 1 |

## STAGE 1
### Mobility Exercises

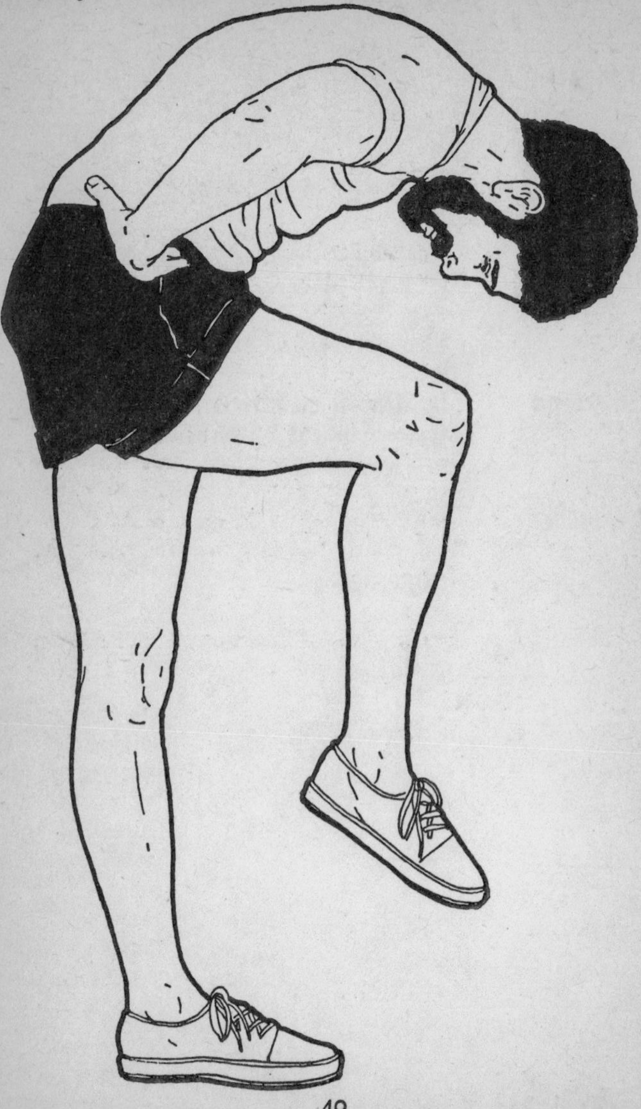

| | |
|---|---|
| Exercise 3 | Trunk, hip and knee bending |
| Purpose | To mobilize the hip and spinal joints; to give greater freedom in forward bending |
| Start | Stand erect, hands on hips |
| Movement | Raise the left knee, at the same time round the spine and bring the forehead down to meet the knee at belt level. Return to the upright position and repeat with other leg. Supporting leg should not be held stiff, bend it slightly, this reduces the pull on the lower back |
| Breathing | Out as you bend and in as you return to the starting position |
| Repetitions | As Exercise 1 |

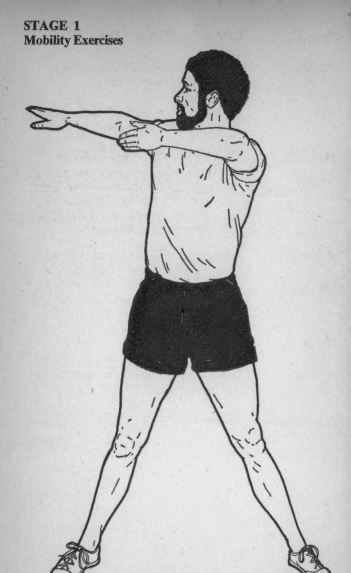

| Exercise 4 | Head, arms and trunk rotating |
|---|---|
| Purpose | To mobilize the spinal joints; to improve the ability to turn the trunk |
| Start | Feet very wide apart, hands outstretched forwards in front of the shoulders |
| Movement | Keep the pelvis and thighs quite still throughout the following movement. Turn the head, shoulders and arms round to the left – let the right elbow bend across the chest. Then turn to the right side bending the left elbow as it crosses the chest |
| Breathing | Breathe freely |
| Repetitions | As Exercise 1 |

The gate

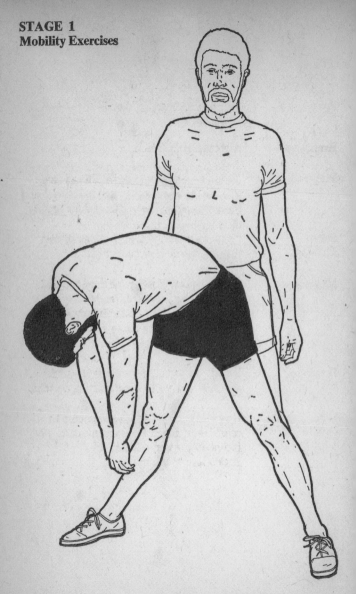

| | |
|---|---|
| Exercise 5 | Alternate ankle reach |
| Purpose | To improve the combined ability to turn, twist and bend the spine, and to stretch the hamstrings (muscles at rear of thigh) gently |
| Start | Feet very wide apart, both palms against the front of the upper left thigh |
| Movement | Let the weight of the trunk bend forwards and downwards towards the left thigh, sliding the hands down the leg towards the left ankle. Return to starting position and repeat to the other side |
| Breathing | Breathe out as the spine bends forwards and in as you return to the starting position |
| Note | No attempt should be made to exceed a comfortable range of movement or to increase the speed – Relax Repetitions as Exercise 1 |

# STAGE 1
## Strength Exercises

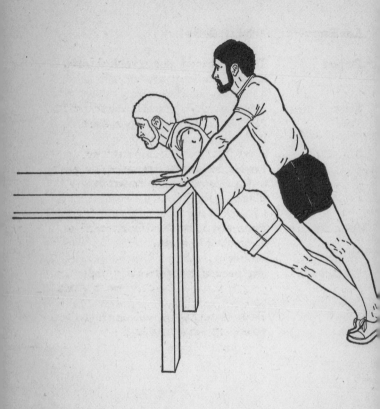

| | |
|---|---|
| Arm Exercise 1 | Table press-ups |
| Purpose | To strengthen and develop arm, shoulder and chest muscles |
| Start | Place both hands on a table, shoulder width apart, body straight, feet 10 in. apart |
| Movement | Allow the chest to touch the table by bending both arms. Immediately straighten both arms and return to the starting position |
| Breathing | Breathe out as you bend the arms and in as you straighten them |
| Repetitions | Begin with a few repetitions (5) and progress over the weeks to between 15 and 30<br>For weak arms place hands on a higher object – or wall at chest level |

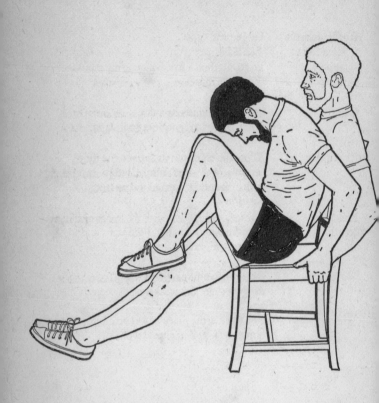

| | |
|---|---|
| Abdominal Exercise 1 | Seated knees up |
| Purpose | To strengthen the tummy muscles |
| Start | Sit on the front edge of a chair, lean back and grip the sides of the chair for control |
| Movement | Raise both knees up towards the chest, allowing the back to bend and permit head to fall forward. Lower and repeat |
| Breathing | Breathe out as you raise the knees and in as you lower |
| Repetitions | As Exercise 1<br>For weak abdominals. Raise alternate leg |

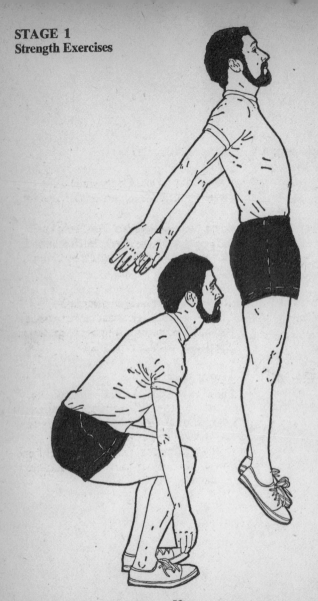

| | |
|---|---|
| Leg Exercise 1 | Jump up from crouch |
| Purpose | Mainly for leg and hip strength. To improve the efficiency of the heart and lungs |
| Start | Feet a few inches apart. Bend both knees until finger tips can reach the floor outside the feet. Allow the heels to come off the floor |
| Movement | Extend the legs and jump vertically upwards. Jump lightly and do not attempt to reach maximum height until experienced, then jump as high as possible |
| Breathing | Breathe freely |
| Repetitions | Start with 10 small jumps and increase over the weeks to 15 to 30 higher jumps in groups of 5 repetitions<br>For weak legs start with half knee bend and hands just past the knees. Do not leap too vigorously |

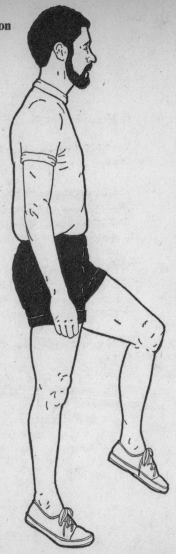

| | |
|---|---|
| Exercise 1 | Running on the spot |
| Purpose | To improve the function of the heart and lungs |
| Start | Standing arms loosely by sides. When running on the spot do not begin by lifting the knees and feet high. As you become fitter, raise the knees higher |
| Movement | Start with very little effort so that you can run on the spot for 30 seconds |
| Breathing | Breathe freely |
| Time | Build up over a long period to 5 or 6 minutes |

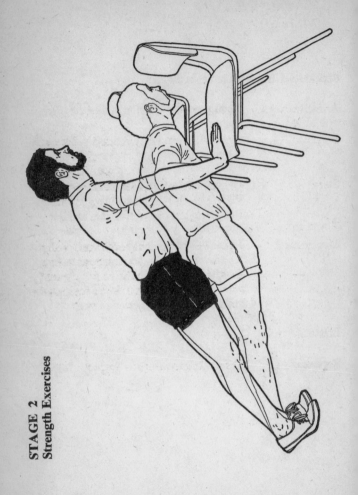

Repeat Mobility exercises as in Stage 1

| | |
|---|---|
| Arm Exercise 2 | Chair press-ups |
| Purpose | As for table press-ups in Stage 1, Strength Exercise 1 |
| Start | Use two chairs, shoulder breadth apart. Place the palm of each hand on a chair. Body straight; toes of both feet on floor |
| Movement | Lower body by bending both arms so that the chest comes to a position approaching the space between the chairs. For the really strong, allow the chest to lower between the chairs |
| Breathing | Freely |
| Repetitions | As for table press-ups in Stage 1 |

## STAGE 2
## Strength Exercises

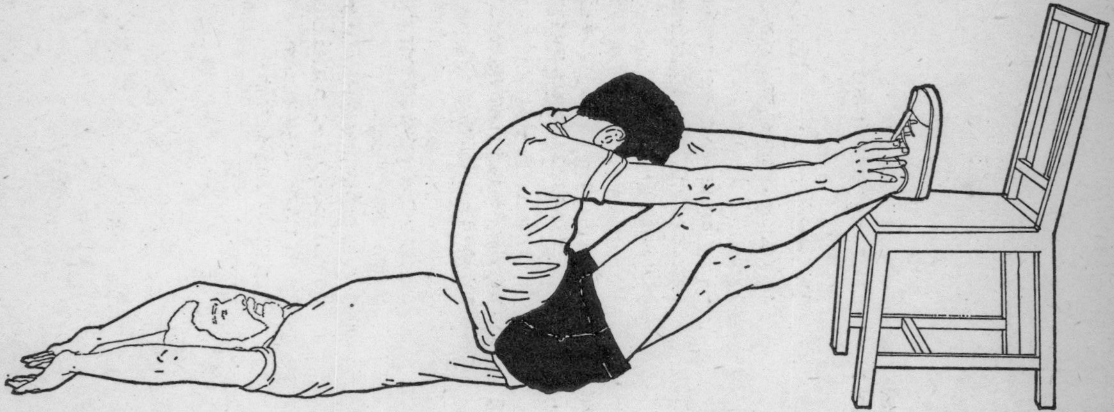

| | |
|---|---|
| Abdominal<br>  Exercise 2 | Chair support V sit-ups |
| Purpose | To develop strength and firmness of the<br>abdominal muscles, and trim the waist-line |
| Start | Back lying on floor, heels resting on front<br>edge of chair. Arms outstretched backwards<br>behind the head |
| Movement | Swing up and forwards to touch the ankles<br>with both hands. Return to start and repeat |
| Breathing | Breathe out as you sit up, in as you return<br>to starting position |
| Repetitions | 8 to 12 times; progress over the weeks to 15<br>to 30 times or more.<br>For the unfit – legs on floor, feet fixed.<br>For the really fit – repeat this exercise after<br>a brief rest after 30 seconds. Two thirds of<br>the previous repetitions |

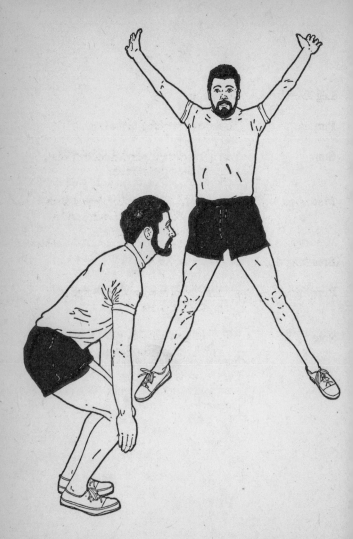

| | |
|---|---|
| Leg Exercise 2 | Star jumps |
| Purpose | To develop strength in the legs |
| Start | Feet a few inches apart, knees half bent, hands by the sides of knees |
| Movement | Leap upwards, feet astride, arm sideways but higher than shoulder level. Land in starting position and repeat |
| Breathing | Freely throughout |
| Repetitions | 10 times. Progress slowly as Stage 1, Strength Exercise 3 |
| Note | Land lightly on the toe, quickly give at the knee to take the shock of landing |

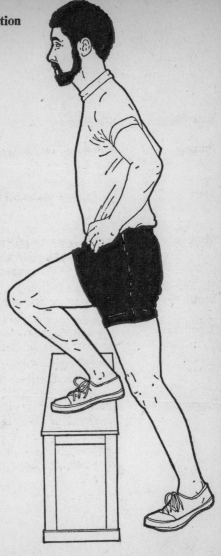

| Exercise 2 | Step ups |
|---|---|
| Purpose | To develop heart and lung efficiency and general fitness |
| Start | Take a low box or stool and stand 12 in. away |
| Movement | Step up first with the left foot leading followed by the right foot. Step down with the left followed by the right |
| Breathing | Breathe freely throughout |
| Repetitions | 15 times with the left foot leading and the same with the right. Add one step each foot, each exercise period until you are stepping up 30 times with each foot |
| Progression | After a few weeks of maximum repetitions increase the height of the box or stool – not to exceed chair height<br>Eventually change from repetitions to a time base as in Stage 1, Light Endurance Exercise 1 |

## STAGE 3
### Strength Exercises

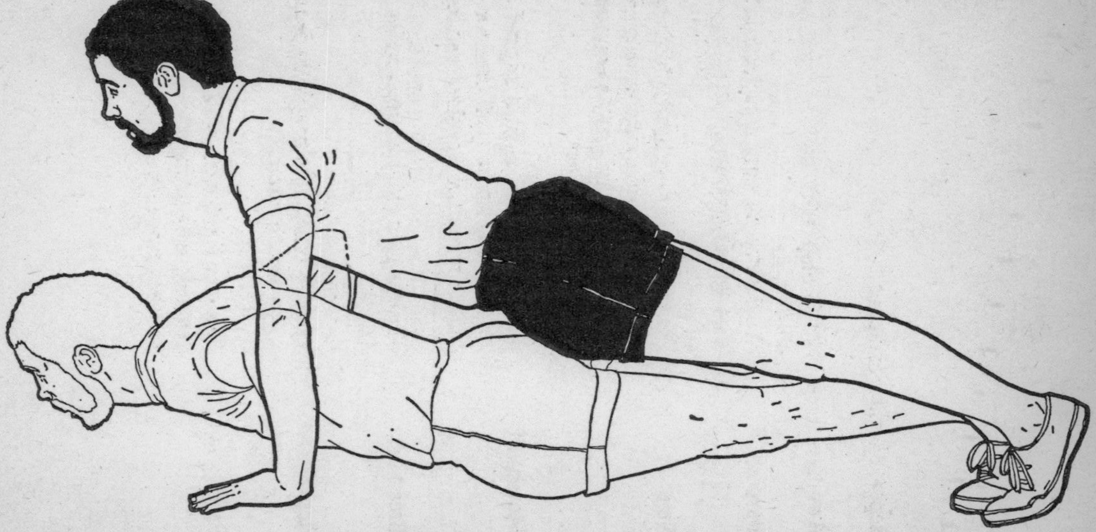

Repeat Mobility exercises as Stage 1.

| Arm Exercise 3 | Floor press-ups |
|---|---|
| Purpose | To develop the same muscles as in Stage 1, Strength Exercise 1 |
| Start | Body straight, both hands placed on floor, fingers pointing forwards and shoulder width apart; feet slightly apart, toes turn in, body resting on floor |
| Movement | Keeping the body rigid, straighten both arms to clear the body off the floor. Lower the body to starting position and repeat |
| Breathing | Breathe in as you press up, and out as you lower |
| Repetitions | 10 to 15 times. Add one, when possible, up to 30 times or more |
| Progression | You can, if you wish, work to reach 30 repetitions by taking a brief rest (30 seconds) two-thirds of the way through |

## STAGE 3
## Strength Exercises

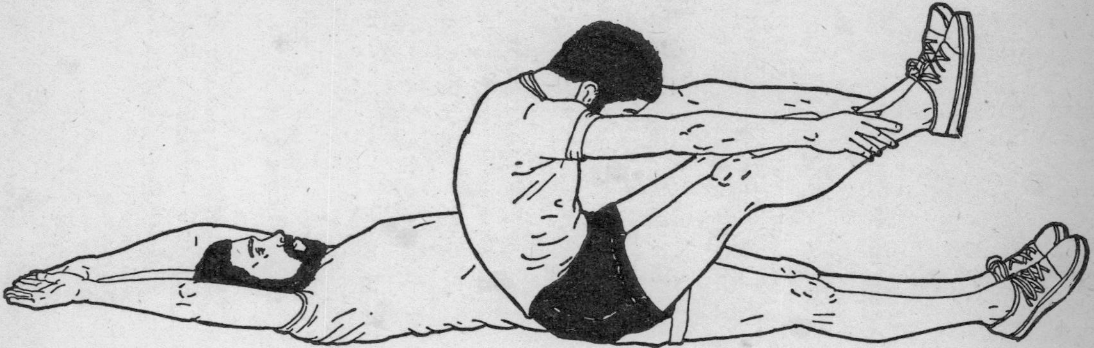

| | |
|---|---|
| Abdominal Exercise 3 | V-sit ups |
| Purpose | To develop strength and trim the mid section |
| Start | Back lying, hands reaching backwards behind the head, toes pointed |
| Movement | Swing into the V-sit position by lifting trunk and legs together so that you balance on both hips. Reach for the ankles with both hands |
| Repetitions | 8 to 12 times; progress over the weeks to 15 to 30 times or more. If you wish to exceed 30 times take a 30 second pause, continue for the additional repetitions |

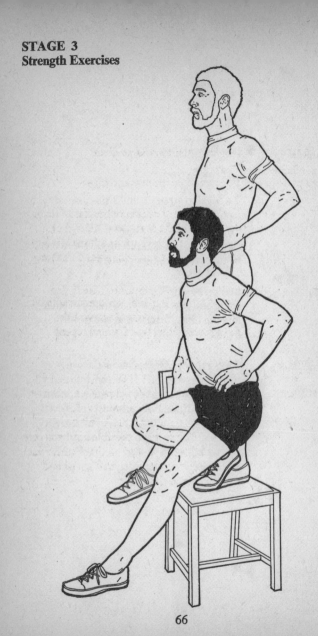

| | |
|---|---|
| Leg Exercise 3 | One leg squat on stool or chair |
| Purpose | To strengthen the legs and hips |
| Start | Take a strong chair. Place the right foot on the middle of the seat. Bend the right leg until you are squatting low, lift the left leg and stretch out straight in front. Hand on back of chair |
| Movement | Straighten the leg until you are standing at your full height, balanced on one foot. Return to starting position and repeat |
| Breathing | Breathe freely throughout |
| Repetitions | Perform a few times with each leg; change from left to right when tired. As follows: 4 left 4 right, 3 left 3 right, 2 left 2 right. Add repetitions when possible until you can perform three groups of 10 times with each leg. You can begin with a half knee bend and assist with the arm |

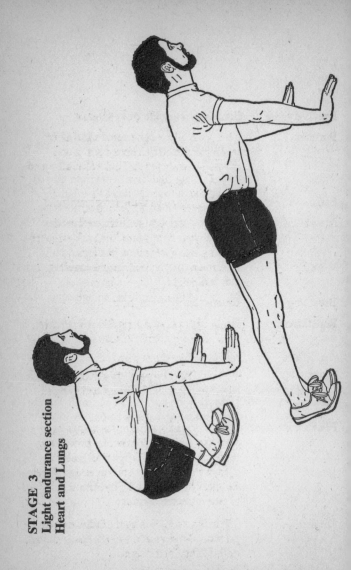

**STAGE 3**
**Light endurance section**
**Heart and Lungs**

| | |
|---|---|
| Exercise 3 | Standing, crouch to front support |
| Purpose | This is a really tough exercise and after several weeks on Schemes 1 and 2 you should be ready for it. To develop all round fitness |
| Start | Standing, arms hanging loosely by sides |
| Movement | Bend knees; put both hands on floor in front of your feet; jump feet back, support body straight, weight on hands and feet. Return to crouch position and stand up. Repeat |
| Breathing | Breathe freely throughout |
| Repetitions | Begin with 15. Add repetitions whenever possible. Aim later to complete 40 or 50 times |
| Note | You can begin by placing both hands on a stout chair or stool before progressing to hand on the floor |
| *Final Comments:* | Do not progress too fast. Remain at each stage for several weeks before proceeding to the next scheme. When you finally change stages, always start at an easy level. Reach and remain at the level most suitable to your personal comfort |
| *Ladies:* | There is no reason why the ladies cannot perform Stages 1 and 2 or the easy version of the difficult exercises |

## Weight training

Don't be alarmed. We are not for a minute suggesting that you should start heaving into the air anything remotely like the massive weights you see Olympic weight-lifters using. It's just that if you have progressed to the stage where you begin to find the previous exercises too light to keep your pulse rate in the target range, then you need to make a choice. Either you are ready to put down this book and go off to take up your favourite sport, relying on that to increase your fitness further, or you need to start working against gradually increasing resistance such as weights can most conveniently provide.

To start you off, and tide you over until your next birthday when someone might be so impressed with your improved shape and general well-being that they insist on buying you proper weight training equipment, we suggest using two cylindrical or waisted plastic bottles, such as washing-up liquid or toilet cleansing solutions come in. As long as you can grasp them comfortably, and they have secure tops, preferably of the screw type to stop the contents shooting out over the bedroom carpet, any convenient size will do. If you begin with them filled with water, at a later stage their weight can be roughly doubled by using sand. This brings the weight of an average sized container up from just over two to well over four pounds or, for those who like to shop in the common market, from one up to two kilos.

Armed with a suitably loaded bottle in each hand, and having warmed up with the first group of mobility exercises, you are ready to practise the five basic weight training movements. This group of relatively advanced exercises should not be introduced into your schedule until you have had several weeks of training on the previous exercises. Also, the same safety

70

rules for limiting the intensity of your exertion according to pulse rate, and the avoidance of distress, apply with more and not less importance while training with weights. Bear in mind that we are not addressing these cautionary words to fit, young athletes, but to the middle 90% of the middle aged and older age groups. This strengthening medicine is strong stuff, so take care not to over-dose yourself.

Well, after all that, we hope we haven't kept you waiting too long to begin wielding your weights. Start with:

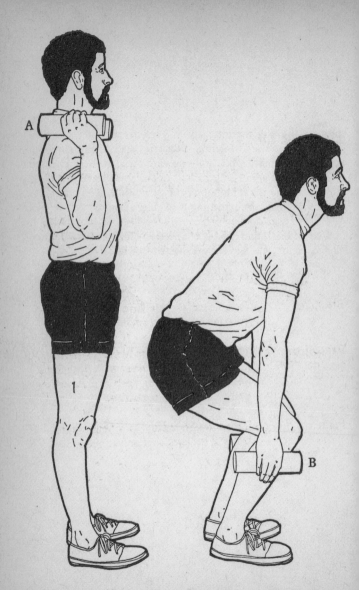

## 1. POWER LIFTS

Start
: Stand erect, feet slightly apart, bottles at side of both shoulders (A)

Movement
: Bend both knees, tilt body forward, keep the back flat but not vertical (the head up and looking forward), lower the bottles to side of calf muscles (B), return immediately to starting position (A)

Breathing
: Breathe out as you bend your knees, in as you stand erect and lift

Repetitions
: Begin with 15 repetitions and proceed by adding 5 repetitions every week, providing you are exercising regularly 3 times weekly, until you reach 30 repetitions

Purpose
: To improve heart and lung fitness and to exercise the legs, back and arm muscles

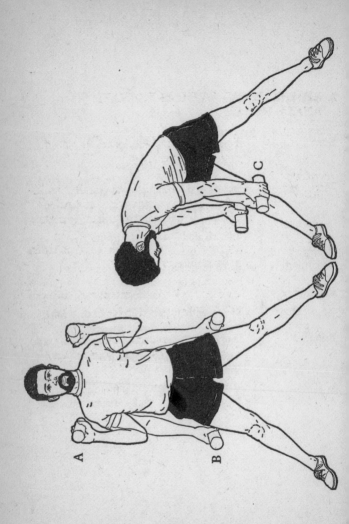

74

# 2. ARM BENDING WITH ALTERNATE ANKLE REACH

Start

Feet wide astride, bottles held at side of each shoulder as (A)

Movement

Lower bottles to side of thighs (B), then to left ankle (C), return directly to starting position (A). Repeat towards other ankle

Breathing

Out as you lower the trunk forwards and in as you return to the start

Repetitions

As Exercise 1. One count for each time you return to the starting position

Purpose

To improve the heart and lung fitness and to exercise the hip, back, waist and arm muscles

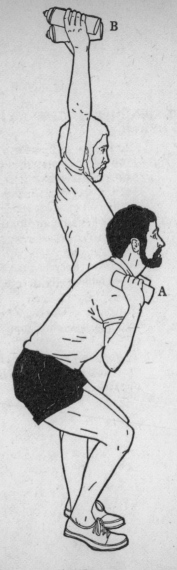

## 3. HEAVE OVERHEAD

Start            Heels a few inches apart and on a four by
                 two inch thick piece of wood or two books
                 of equal thickness, bottles held at the side
                 of each shoulder, eyes looking forward (A)

Movement         Heave bottles to arms' length overhead (B)
                 by extending the arms and legs together;
                 return to start (A)

Breathing        Breathe in as you heave overhead and out
                 as you bend the knees

Repetitions      As Exercise 1

Purpose          To improve the heart and lung fitness, and
                 to exercise the leg, hip, back and arms and
                 shoulders

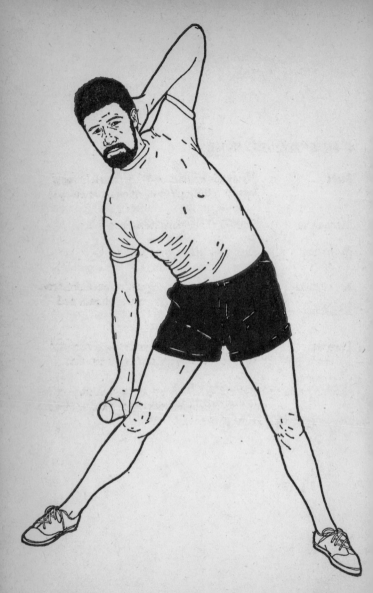

## 4. SIDE TO SIDE BENDS

Start            Feet wide astride, bottle in the right hand
                 by side of thigh, left hand behind neck (A)

Movement         Bend as far as possible to each side

Breathing        Freely throughout

Repetitions      As Exercise 1. One repetition each time you
                 return to position (A), change hands and
                 repeat

Purpose          To improve the heart and lung fitness and
                 to exercise the spine and waist muscles

(At this point repeat running on the spot for 3–5 minutes from
your present schedule in the light endurance section, before
proceeding with your next exercise.)

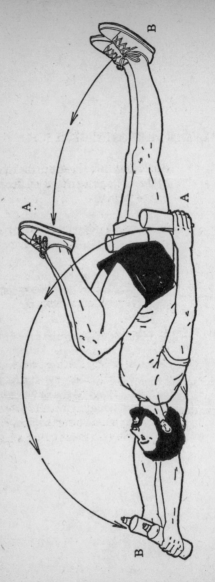

## 5. BACK LYING AND ARM STRETCH

Start                 Back lying, knees bend up on to chest, arms
                      by the side, bottles resting on floor by the
                      side of thighs.

Movement              Reach backwards with the arms in a half
                      circle, at the same time stretch the legs into
                      position (B)

Breathing             Out as you flex the thighs on to the chest,
                      and in as you stretch into (B)

Repetitions           As Exercise 1

Purpose               To mobilize the chest cage and to exercise
                      the abdominals, chest and shoulder muscles
                      these weight training exercises with bottles
                      are merely an introduction to proper weight
                      training with the correct equipment for
                      people who wish to exercise at a higher level

*How can you judge your progress?*

Rewards for our efforts is one of the most strongly motivating factors in life, and exercise training is no exception. If we can measure the increasing amount of physical work we can do in a given time and for a given pulse rate, then we are likely to continue or even increase our efforts. Some would describe this as being a bio-feedback system with positive entropy. Others would simply say it's nice to know where you are.

Either way, there are several methods of judging your progress. One is to count the total number of movements done during the exercise periods. You can make this a more exact method of rating the intensity of the work by scoring each exercise according to the weights if any used. You will find as you become fitter that you can work faster and take shorter and shorter rests, so that whatever your scale of exercise, the amount you can do increases, often by a surprisingly large amount.

Another way of measuring your increasing fitness is to take your pulse at the start and finish of your schedule, and add these two values together. This way you will also find after a few months of regular training, not only that you have a slower resting heart rate, but that both during and after exercise your heart is beating more slowly and working more efficiently at a given intensity of exercise.

The rate at which your heart slows down again after exercise is another good guide to progress. You can try periodically taking your pulse rate immediately after finishing the last exercise in the schedule, and then again 90 seconds later. The fall in rate in this limited period is likely to get considerably greater as you get fitter showing your more rapid recovery from exertion.

Whichever method you use, we feel sure that you will find encouraging proof that your heart and lungs have become much more efficient in dealing with physical effort, and that you will be recovering faster afterwards. These rewards will go a long way to convince you of the value of exercise and motivate you to continue with your programme.

You may also like to turn, bend and twist in the early days and later take the same measurements again. This should demonstrate your increasing suppleness in the form of greater mobility through several ranges of movement.

Lastly, if you are overweight, have a tyre check. Pinch up between the thumb and fore-finger the skin and fat over the side of your mid-riff. If it is over half an inch thick then you need to continue to restrict the sugar and starch in your diet as well as keeping on with the exercise. Even that too solid flesh will yield to the combined attack of both measures, given the will to go on.

# CHAPTER SIX

# WHERE

*Where do these principles apply to other forms of exercise?*

There are many different roads to fitness. What we have tried to do in the other chapters is to distil from over ten years experience with unfit adults at the City Gymnasium, the essence of exercise. Like other distillates such as whisky, this is strong stuff and needs to be taken in small doses. However weak your flesh, we hope the resulting spirit will see you well along the path to fitness.

As well as describing these essential ingredients of exercising in safety and comfort, this book gives you some starting schedules to carefully and progressively increase your mobility, strength and endurance until a basic level of fitness is reached. Now you are ready for the more advanced and vigorous forms of exercise. One which is conveniently packaged and can be carried out at home is the 'condensed recipe' weight training course described in the previous chapter. Using this system it is possible to stay really fit with only a 15 to 20 minutes exercise period two or three times each week.

The same principles, however, apply to other forms of exercise, and many people will only see the starting schedules as a means to an end, the end being their favourite form of sport. It's worth going over these principles again before seeing where they apply to other forms of exercise.

Firstly, unless you want to give up work and just spend most of your day exercising, the exercise needs to be vigorous enough to give you maximum benefit in minimum time. It should, however, not be violent or consist of maximal efforts, where you strain like hell and get nowhere. This form of exercise, where the load on the muscles is too great to be moved and the tension in the muscle increases because it does not shorten or lengthen, is called isometric (iso = same, metric = length). It has the disadvantages that it pushes up the blood pressure, and slows the flow of blood back to the heart. It is the type of effort involved in pushing your car up a hill, straining to lift an impossibly heavy weight, or pulling on a cork-screw when the cork won't shift. All these supreme efforts are bad for the heart, back and mind alike, when really unfit.

The preferable type of exercise is one where the muscles are free to move because the load on them is moderate or light. Then the tension or tone in them stays about the same, which is known as isotonic exercise (iso = same, tonic = tone). This allows the blood to flow easily through the muscles, improves the return of blood to the heart, and raises the blood pressure by little or nothing. It also doesn't cause muscle cramps or strains, which adds to your comfort during and after exercise.

A gradual build-up in the intensity of exercise is also desirable, even when you have prepared your body for some months previously with the basic course described here. This may be difficult to achieve, particularly in competitive sports, which tend to be all or nothing events. The 'death or glory' approach to sport is really not recommended if you are a previously unfit person of over 30. Keep your competitive instincts under control, and never be too proud to say you've had enough. Don't flog yourself until you drop, or it might be permanent!

Similarly, you won't be able to do the same amount of exercise every week, all the year round. Everyone has quite large variations in physical condition, mood and energy levels. Let your pulse rate and the way you feel when you exercise be your guide. You will soon know when you are doing too much as you learn to control the intensity and amount of exertion with these simple but vitally important measures.

Suggestions about mid-morning or before lunch being the best time for exercise also apply, particularly to the more strenuous forms of sport. Monday to Friday, however, you may have to settle for the early morning session for doing the home-based exercises. These are particularly useful, not only as a way of getting ready to take up your sport of choice, but also to keep you fit 'out of season'.

Keeping warm, but not getting over-heated, is also important for all forms of exercise. Obviously, if your surroundings are cold, you will need a warm track suit. This is not just a luxury – it is a necessity. Preferably, however, your surroundings should be comfortably warm, and then you will need shorts and singlet. As comfort and what the French call 'esprit de corps' or, in psychologists' jargon, 'body-image', play a large part in helping you to enjoy exercise, it's worth spending a reasonable amount to get the 'right' gear. Shoes that don't fit, baggy below-knee shorts of ancient cut, and a shirt where the sleeves fall over the wrist and the collar strangles you, don't look or feel inspiring, and hide rather than display the magnificent physique which is developing beneath them.

Also, for most forms of exercise which are sufficiently vigorous to bring you to even a moderate level of fitness, you need to 'get a glow on'. Translated into more realistic terms, this means you need to perspire freely or even, to put it bluntly, sweat. Washable sports kit and some form of bathing or showering facilities are therefore highly desirable if *you* wish to remain desirable.

Some people like to increase the sweating rate still further by taking a sauna after exercise. While many people feel much better after a sauna, it is a poor substitute for exercise. Also, research carried out at the City Gymnasium has shown that the rapid heart rate and profound fall in blood pressure which result from prolonging a really hot sauna bath for much more than five minutes, may well place a considerable strain on the unfit heart. Having a cold shower after a sauna, however stimulating it may be, is a variety of circulatory gymnastics which is not recommended.

This brings us to our last general point which is that just as maximum benefit from exercise comes on within two to three months of starting, so most wears off within two to three months of stopping. Therefore exercise needs to be more than an occasional fling. It needs to become a regular part of your way of life. This is an additional reason for making exercise physically and emotionally attractive. Variety is the spice of exercise, so that a fitness programme which concentrates on just one form of activity, such as a static bicycle or rowing machine, not only develops just a few muscle groups, but tends rapidly to become monotonous so that after a few weeks or months you give up. Music can do much to add interest to your indoor schedules, but you shouldn't necessarily let it impose its own tempo on your movements. Sport has its own built-in variety, as each game is different and if interest lags you can always stop and have a chat with the people you are playing with.

Let's have a look at different forms of physical activity and the ways in which these general principles apply to them.

*Pedestrian pastimes*

Walking, as we have already said, is a good way of taking the first steps towards getting fit. It can also be made very gently progressive by increasing pace, distance and gradient. However, unless you have a steep hill at least a mile long with a prevailing head wind blowing down it right on your door step, it is unlikely that walking on its own will provide the intensity of exercise needed to keep you fully fit.

Failing this, you will need to jog or run to get further on your fitness plan. Given the same attention to pulse rates, avoidance of discomfort and extreme cold, and preliminary weight reduction in the very obese, either can be a very good form of exercise. A good safety rule is never to jog or run at a pace which would make it difficult to talk to someone going along with you. Not that we suggest you should talk much on the way round, as it is likely to spoil your concentration and make your breathing erratic. Again, avoid competition, especially with younger, fitter people, as you are likely to drive yourself too hard, and override warning symptoms of fatigue.

*Cycling*

Cycling has a great deal to recommend it as a way of getting fit. Firstly, it is the right type of smooth, regular, rhythmic, non-maximal or, in other words, 'isotonic' exercise. Providing he has taken some notice of the advice given several times previously in this book, and does not begin cycling up the steepest hill he can find in bottom gear just to prove his determination to do it if it kills him, which it might, the cyclist can progress in easy stages from a very low to quite a high level of fitness. Even the very overweight individual can start straight in on cycling as his weight is supported.

Secondly, it is one of the most intense forms of exercise which can be taken without the need to change clothing. This is because, given the right type of clothing with reasonable ventilation, the rate of flow of air over the body is sufficient to evaporate the perspiration as it forms, so that the cyclist remains socially acceptable and cool. The amount of time spent travelling to or changing for other forms of exercise is often considerably greater than the exercise period itself.

Thirdly, commuting by bicycle means that you not only save a rapidly increasing amount of money and lessen the frustrations of rush-hour travel to the point where it becomes a positive pleasure to go to work, but you also don't have to take time off during the day or at the weekend to exercise. This factor of it being built into your everyday life is very important as it means that you are more likely to keep it up because it is both functional and enjoyable, as well as keeping you fit.

The main disadvantage of cycling, and the one which puts many people off, is the danger of an accident. The complete lack of cycling facilities in most of our major cities, particularly in the form of separate safe cycle-ways, seems a great pity, especially when for a relatively small financial outlay, and with a few changes in the bye-laws regarding the use of parks and paths for cycling, the situation could be greatly improved. This would simultaneously benefit both the health and temper of the people enticed out of their tin coffins on wheels.

## Swimming

This is another excellent form of exercise, which can bring you gradually to a very high level of fitness providing you really train and don't just float about and paddle. This can be difficult in public pools, especially when they are crowded with children: there may be a need for special times or separate lanes for serious swimmers doing their daily dozen lengths.

The advantages of swimming are many. Not only is the intensity of exercise easily variable, it is the type of smooth, rhythmic, isotonic exercise which gives the least strain and most gain. Even more than with cycling, the entire body weight is supported, so that the very overweight individual is at no disadvantage in this situation, and may even do better than his lean fellow-swimmer by floating higher in the water. Certainly he will be better insulated, although even at the comfortable temperature of most indoor pools, additional fat is being burned up to maintain body temperature. Really cold conditions, although the delight of some fresh air fanatics, probably because of the surge of the kick hormone, noradrenaline, which a cold plunge produces, are best avoided by the less hardy swimming novices. It takes an ardent thermal masochist to really benefit from a prolonged steam heat sauna or icy dip, and particularly one followed immediately by the other. Surviving this combination is a good test of your heart and blood vessels, but probably does little to improve their condition.

The safety of swimming under ordinary indoor conditions is illustrated by the absence of heart attacks during the sponsored swims organized by the British Heart Foundation. In these a large number of very unfit people, many of whom have heart conditions, do several lengths of the pool to raise money for this very worthwhile charity. Often this is the first vigorous exercise they may have taken for several years, and yet to the relief of the organizers they not only survive unharmed, but frequently having 'taken the plunge' continue this very sociable and congenial form of exercise with their families.

*Ball games*

These tend to be erratic and often over-competitive pastimes which can lead to muscle strains, joint sprains and even chest pains. Certainly they are very much safer from all these points of view once you've done the initial course of exercises which this book describes. This will not only have increased your suppleness, strength and stamina, but perhaps more importantly will have given you that body-sense needed to regulate your exertion.

Given the basic rules of exercising safely which we have already described, it is then a matter of what you enjoy. Every sport has something to recommend it, if only that a few people are keen enough to play it. A ball, however, is a symbol of competition in the hunt or aggression in the field. Footballs and tennis balls are either leathery objects or furry objects resembling and often made from the hide of the animals our ancestors used to hunt. Balls to be thrown, like cricket and baseballs, tend to be harder like the stones used to stun the prey.

Except for the running component, in most games striking the ball with the foot, hand, racket or club is insufficient on its own to raise the pulse rate into the optimal zone. Most ball games then resolve themselves into a series of jerky runs punctuated with sudden, vicious, violent jabs with arm or leg. Also, as the aim of games is not as the poem would have it, to play but to win, and speed and co-ordination tend to decrease with age, the natural tendency is for participation in these pastimes to decrease just when, from the health point of view, it starts to be important. Further, the harassed middle-aged businessman and family man seldom has time or inclination to travel many miles across the city in which he lives to take part in such activities. For all these reasons we feel that many business firms and large organizations would do well to invest more money in on-the-spot facilities, such as gymnasia, swimming pools, with squash and badminton courts for those who insist in competing, rather than have large sports fields miles away which only a few already fit and hardened exercise enthusiasts will use.

This change in emphasis in the provision of facilities, we feel, needs to be accompanied by an even greater increase in the number of suitably qualified instructors in adult fitness. Last but not least, we need to know a great deal more about the many different ways of helping all those who would like to enjoy the multiple benefits of fitness. Chief of these is the introduction of a positive rather than a negative approach to living as part of the philosophy of exercise.

*Very large claims are made for this book. Full details of the extensive trials on which it is based are given in the following pages.*

*While the full benefits of the system can be enjoyed without studying these pages, new insights can be derived from an understanding of the principles on which it is based.*

# BRITISH PILOT STUDY OF EXERCISE THERAPY

## 1. Middle-aged men

M. E. Carruthers, M.D., M.R.C.Path.,
Senior Lecturer,
Department of Chemical Pathology (Research)
St. Mary's Hospital Medical School,
London, W2 1PG

R. H. T. Edwards, B.Sc., Ph.D., M.B., M.R.C.P.,
Lecturer and Honorary Consultant Physician
Professor of Metabolic Medicine, University College Hospital,
London WC1

and

N. B. Pride, M.D., F.R.C.P.,
Senior Lecturer and Honorary Consultant Physician,
Department of Medicine, Royal Postgraduate Medical School, W.12.

P. Nixon, F.R.C.P.,
Consultant Cardiologist,
Charing Cross Hospital,
London, W.6.

and

Cecily de Moncheaux, Ph.D.,
Senior Lecturer,
Department of Psychiatry,
University College Hospital,
London, W.C.1.

Exercises designed and supervised
by Alistair Murray, M.S.R.G.,
Director of the City Gym.

To
Denis Howell, Minister of Sport, in gratitude for his
encouragement and support in this research project.

# SUMMARY

*The physiological and biochemical effects of a carefully graduated course of vigorous gymnasium training with two or three weekly exercise sessions lasting only 15 minutes have been studied in middle-aged London business men.*

*Activity diaries and psychological questionnaires indicated that these men had a positive attitude to exercise which was probably greater than average. The gymnasium exercises caused a large oxygen debt and considerable rises in plasma catecholamines and lactate levels. A close correlation was found between the pulse rate during exercise and the Borg scale of perceived exertion, so that both could be used to ensure that short periods of exercise were sufficiently vigorous to produce a training effect, and protect against over-exertion. The acceptability of this particular exercise regime was shown by the low fall-out and injury rate.*

*It is suggested that this exercise training programme possesses many features which are advantageous if increased physical activity is to be more widely used as a method of reducing some of the risk factors in coronary heart disease.*

# INTRODUCTION

*Exercise is now being increasingly recommended, both in its own right as an enjoyable recreational pastime[1] and as a means of preventing some of the diseases associated with urban life, particularly coronary heart disease.[2,3] In view of the current interest in 'exercise therapy', both to prevent and treat coronary disease, we thought it appropriate to report a pilot study of a course of gymnasium training designed to enhance cardiovascular fitness in middle-aged men.*

*There have been several studies of the effects of physical training in middle-aged men, especially in Scandinavia[4-6] and America,[7-10] but no multidisciplinary investigations in this field have been reported in Great Britain. The need for a broadly based approach to such studies is illustrated by the wide range of advantages attributed to exercise listed in Table 1.*

*Ideally, such exercise should be safe, acceptable, fitness-producing and economic. On the basis of 'firstly do no harm', safety must be the overriding factor in advising the unfit adult who wishes to exercise. Acceptability is the next consideration, as the finest schemes are useless if they remain unused. Fitness, in the sense of increased physical well-being, is the aim of most who exercise. Economy is essential for wide acceptance, not only from the financial aspect, but also in terms of the closely related factors of the time and space required.*

*The opportunity to study a form of exercise which appeared to offer many of these features arose in this country from a collaboration between the late Dr. Harold Lewis of the Medical Research Council and Mr. Alistair Murray, Director of the City Gymnasium in London.*

## SUBJECTS

*The study group consisted of a total of 302 men, mean age 37 years (range 26–57), with no history of cardiac disease, who had enrolled at the Gymnasium for a course of physical training.*

94

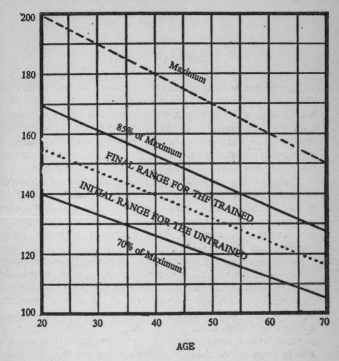

Fig. 1. *Pulse rate ranges for healthy men at different stages of gymnasium training*

95

For ethical reasons the General Practitioner's consent had to be obtained in writing before individuals could take part in the study, even though they were participating fully in gymnasium activities. This often delayed the initial investigations for several weeks, during which time a considerable 'training' effect became apparent. Also, as these individuals were paying standard fees, it was found to be difficult to raise the question of time-consuming and mildly inconvenient research procedures in the early weeks without putting the more nervous of them off the idea of exercise altogether. There was thus an unintended bias towards selection of the more robust and less anxious individuals, and towards those who had already attended the Gymnasium for several weeks.

## THE EXERCISE PROGRAMME

The exercise programme used was a carefully graded course of physical training designed by Mr. Alistair Murray. Each person exercised for 15 minute periods two or three times each week, starting at very low work rates, and frequently monitoring his own pulse rate to ensure that it remained within the predetermined limits (fig. 1). The rhythmic submaximal movements were predominantly isotonic rather than isometric in character,[12] light weight loading being introduced only gradually and carefully in relation to observed progress to maintain the training effect of a short period of exertion. In addition to 'free' exercises, adjustable weight training equipment was used, and the intensity of the exercise increased by weight increments of just 2–3 lbs, using a formula involving the product of repetitions and resistance in pounds (Repounds). This exercise intensity score (Repounds) enabled work rates to be replicated, increased or decreased, and quantitatively related to changes in physiological and biochemical variables. The City Gymnasium Programme consisted of 10 varied movements, closely approaching the ideal of whole-body exercise, and avoiding the monotony inherent in training limited muscle groups, e.g. on a stationary bicycle.

A psychophysical scale comprising equal intervals from 6 to 20 was used to rate perceived exertion.[13] Values on this scale when multiplied by 10 are known to correspond closely with the exercise heart rate and this was found to be the case during most of the vigorous exercise period (fig. 2).

## PHYSIOLOGICAL STUDIES

The exercise intensity scores achieved at each session in the Gymnasium showed large and progressive rises over a six-month period (fig. 3). The 40 men exercising three times each week showed

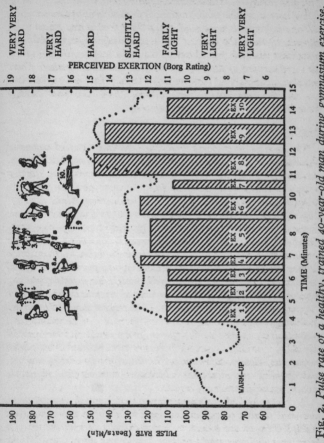

Fig. 2. Pulse rate of a healthy, trained 40-year-old man during gymnasium exercise, showing correlation with mean ratings of perceived exertion in 13 men

97

*a larger increase ($p < 0.001$) than a group of 30 attending twice a week. These results imply considerable rises in effort capacity at a given pulse rate, as only a slight increase in exercise pulse rate was allowed in the training programme.*

The oxygen uptake during a standard schedule of the 10 exercises was studied at the Gymnasium in 13 healthy men aged between 26 and 53 years (mean 37 years), with an average height of 175·7 cm (range 168·0–185·7 cm) and weight of 80·4 kg (range 66·0–106·2 kg). Body fat, estimated from skinfold thickness measurements, amounted to 19·5% of body weight (range 12·5–27·3). Resting pulse rate averaged 65 beats/min (range 52–88) and mean resting blood pressure was 124/78 mm Hg (systolic range 165–95, diastolic range 90–52). Mean resting oxygen uptake ($\dot{V}O_2$) measured by a Douglas bag technique was 310 ml/min (range 235–409 ml/min). Subjects then performed the standard schedule of 10 exercises, completed on average in 10 minutes (range 7½–12 minutes). Oxygen uptake was measured over the whole exercise period and again during 10 minutes of recovery in the supine position. Exercise intensity score varied widely in the different subjects, the average being 6920 'Repounds'/min (range 3870–10520), i.e. rather higher than the average for a larger group in fig. 3. Exercise oxygen uptake averaged 1750 ml/min (range 1340–2140), equivalent to 21·9 ml kg/min (range 15·2–28·2), and it was estimated that this represented 50–65% of the maximum $\dot{V}O_2$. Exercise intensity score correlated significantly with oxygen uptake ($r = 0.64$). This correlation was improved by relating the score to excess oxygen uptake, i.e. exercise $\dot{V}O_2$ minus that at rest ($r = 0.78$). The oxygen debt averaged 3·5 litres (S.D. ±1·7).

Another group of 19 healthy men, mean age 44·5 years (range 35–54) were studied during an increasing work rate test[14] on a cycle ergometer. These studies were performed in the exercise laboratory at the Royal Postgraduate Medical School, Hammersmith Hospital, on four occasions, twice during their first week of involvement in the study, which was often their second or third week of training, and again eight and 14 weeks later. The test was stopped when heart rate reached 85% of the maximum value predicted from the subject's age (fig. 1). Two periods of submaximal exercise (300 and 600 kpm/min, 50 and 100 watts respectively) were also performed and ventilation ($\dot{V}E$), oxygen uptake ($\dot{V}O_2$) and heart rate measured.

The results of the cycle ergometer tests are shown in Table II, with cardiac frequencies and ventilation interpolated to oxygen intakes of 1·0 and 1·5 litres/min. At the initial assessment the values of cardiac frequency and ventilation at standard oxygen intakes were

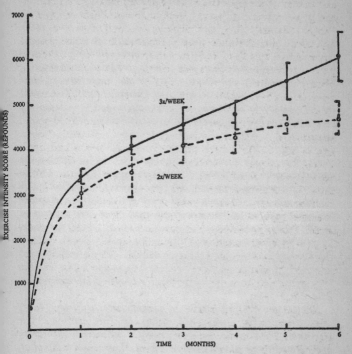

Fig. 3. *Mean (±S.E.) increase in exercise intensity score with length of gymnasium training for 40 men exercising three times each week, compared with 30 men exercising twice weekly*

*similar to those found previously for non-athletic middle-aged men.*[14],[15] *Repeat studies after a further eight and 14 weeks of the Gymnasium programme showed no significant changes in heart rate or ventilatory response during exercise. Thus, despite the improved ability to perform the Gymnasium exercises, no improvement in performance was demonstrated on the cycle ergometer.*

## HABITUAL ACTIVITY STUDY

*Especially designed diary cards*[16] *were issued to 40 volunteers who recorded details of their activities during three consecutive working days and weekends. These cards were analysed according to whether the subject worked in the 'City' or was employed elsewhere. The results of the analysis are shown in Tables III and IV. There is considerable variation in the activity pattern and an unexpected finding was the large amount of time spent walking by both groups.*

## PSYCHOLOGICAL STUDY

*The aim of the psychological study was to characterize the individuals with variables which might subsequently prove valuable in cross-disciplinary analyses of data on exercise therapy effects. The psychological findings summarized below are descriptive, enabling comparison of the Gymnasium group with other UK samples of similar age and social status.*

*Three variables were investigated:*

*1. Long-term personality pattern*

*2. Current emotional status*

*3. History of recent life events*

*Subjects were sent a 5-day kit of questionnaires which they filled in anonymously and posted to the investigator. Fifty-one out of the 61 volunteers completed the assignment. Their ages ranged from 26–61 years (mean 39 years).*

*1.* Personality patterns

*(a)* Extraversion-introversion[17]

*The test includes items designed to characterize the high sociability, liking for activity and impulsiveness of the extrovert, in contrast to reservation, tendency to shyness and self-control of the introvert. Scores for our sample gave a mean $11\cdot60\pm3\cdot84$ ($n = 47$), values which are very close to those for matched groups of normal UK males.*

*(b)* Hostility *was assessed by the use of the Hostility and Direction of Hostility Questionnaire.*[18] *For 'general hostility' our sample gave*

*a mean of 15·28 ± 5·69 (n = 46), slightly but not significantly above the values they published for other normal groups. The sample proved to be slightly more extrapunitive (mean 1·50 ± 6·29) than normal in direction of hostility.*

*In summary, the personality measures indicated that the sample was fairly typical of a normal population of the same age and socio-economic grouping.*

## 2. Current emotional state

*This was assessed by subjects making a daily check over five days against a list of 55 mood items. The list comprised descriptions of moods and emotions; anger, fear, depression and fatigue, alertness and happiness. As with most normal samples, there was a pre-ponderance of positive over negative affect. Fear was less common than other negative moods in the anger and fatigue groups. The relatively frequency of moods in the active-alert group was higher than in other normal samples, reflecting the 'get up and go' character of the Gymnasium population.*

## 3. History of recent life events

*It seemed to us to be important to investigate the degree of strain under which a man may be living as a consequence of the need to adapt to a high frequency of events in his life, whether these be desired by him or not. A measure originated by Rahe[19] was adapted for use with our sample and consisted of 50 items covering events concerning family, employment, health and finances over three periods in the immediate past: 0–6 months, 7–12 months, 1–2 years. The total number of life events recorded by our subjects for the 2-year period varied widely, from 6 to 40, with a mean of 13·3 ± 7·2. The highest score was in the 0–6 month period, the recency but not the intensity of events affecting their recall. In the absence of compar-ative data from other UK samples, the interest of the life event data residues in its interaction with other variables, e.g. lipid levels, which will be reported later.*

## BIOCHEMICAL STUDIES

*The biochemical methods used were those described by Taggart and Carruthers.[20]*

### (a) Short-term effects

*Blood samples were taken before and within a minute of the end of exercise in 107 volunteers. The results are shown in Table V. Both noradrenaline and adrenaline rose during exercise, the former accounting for most of the increase in total catecholamine level.[21]*

The rise in blood sugar correlated poorly with the increase in adrenaline ($r = 0.206$ $p < 0.05$) while the high post-exercise lactate levels are consistent with the finding of a large oxygen debt. Rises in plasma proteins and cholesterol could be accounted for by haemo-concentration (pcv $40.78 \pm 0.42\%$ pre $42.55 \pm 0.47\%$ pest. $p < 0.001$). Free fatty acid and triglyceride levels remained high but unchanged after exercise. In the presence of increased plasma noradrenaline levels, the constancy of the free fatty acid and triglyceride levels suggest that lipolysis and fatty acid utilization are considerably augmented by this form of exercise.

(b) Long-term effects

In 17 volunteers who continued to attend the Gymnasium regularly, from the fourth month onwards no significant changes were found in any of the 11 biochemical variables listed in Table V as measured serially over a period of up to two years. This confirms the findings reported in the second paper that the maximum change in biochemical and haemodynamic variables is achieved within three months of starting the training programme, and is maintained as long as the subject continues to exercise regularly.

## DISCUSSION

The aim of this study was to characterize in physiological and biochemical terms a system of weight-assisted gymnasium exercises, and to examine the habitual activity and psychology of the middle-aged men who volunteered for this type of training.

The regime at the City Gymnasium was not very demanding physically. Subjects attended two, or more often three times a week, and performed a period of exercise which lasted an average of 15 minutes on each occasion. The work intensity was estimated to represent $50-65\%$ of the individual's maximum oxygen intake. Such a level of exercise, carried out for only 15 minutes two or three times a week, would not be considered on the basis of other studies carried out on fitter and younger people[22] to be sufficient to result in substantial physiological changes. However, Nordesjö,[22] starting with non-athletic students, found a significant training effect with exercise of this intensity, frequency and duration, and that this regime was the most acceptable to those training.

Also, the oxygen debt and increase in blood lactate resulting from the 15 minute period of exercise were larger than would be expected from the oxygen uptake. This may be because some of the exercises carried out in the Gymnasium affect predominantly the arm, shoulder and back muscles, and it is probable that these muscles were *working closer to their maximum capacity than is indicated by measurement of the whole body oxygen intake during exercise. Such considerations may be important in defining the term 'vigorous' in relation to the finding of Morris et al[2] that 'habitual vigorous exercise during leisure time reduces the incidence of coronary heart disease in middle-age among male sedentary workers'.*

*There are two possible explanations for the absence of significant changes in the responses to exercise in the subjects studied at Hammersmith. One is that the particular subjects studied there were already partly trained at the time they were first studied. This is likely in view of the delay in initiating the investigation due to the need to consent from the subjects' General Practitioners. The other is that the training programme involved mainly upper limb and trunk muscle groups not much used in cycling, which therefore showed little change.[24]*

*The psychological characteristics of the Gymnasium population studied were reasonably typical of the male population of the same age, but tended to be slightly more extroverted and to have 'active' rather than 'passive' personalities. This conclusion was supported by the finding that a majority of the subjects who volunteered took part in physically active pursuits, playing golf or squash, swimming, sailing, etc. The measurements made of physical work capacity showed that on average the subjects had a physiological performance similar to that of a moderately active group of the same age.*

*The most important features of this gymnasium-based exercise programme were its acceptability and safety. The proportion of subjects ceasing exercise before their membership subscription lapsed (drop-out rate) was extremely low for unfit adults taking up any form of exercise, averaging 5, 10 and 15% for the two, six and 12 month attenders respectively. This compares favourably with the findings of Sanne and Wilhelmsen[5] who found that 30% dropped out within one year. Less than 2% of the subjects suffered minor injuries sufficient to make them even temporarily cease training. The few injuries that did occur were nearly all transient mild recurrences of pre-existing 'back' troubles.*

*The individual tuition and supervision of progress by the trained remedial gymnasts running the Gymnasium, rather than class exercises, helped to secure an adequate amount of exercise without risk of over-exertion. The need for a considerable margin of safety is emphasized by the tests of cardiac function reported in the second article. The safety of exercise as carried out under these conditions is demonstrated by the fact that although approximately a fifth of the 2,500 people training in the Gymnasium over the past seven years* were known to have cardiovascular disease, none suffered a heart attack whilst exercising.[25] In view of the number of sudden deaths occurring in middle-aged sportsmen during exercise, it is suggested that extremely few physical educationalists or sports coaches are qualified to deal with the unfit adult.[26]

The problems encountered in running this pilot study have mainly been ones of recruitment from a self-selected group of middle-aged men who are less accustomed to taking part in clinical investigations of this type than their counterparts in many Scandinavian countries. Late enrolment made it difficult to chart changes attributable to this scheme which would, in any case, have required a non-exercising control group. This is included in an extension of this study investigating alterations in coronary risk factors over a longer period. Time pressures and travelling difficulties limited the number of volunteers willing to visit other hospitals for the more detailed physiological and cardiological tests. Although the intensity of work as measured by the 'Exercise Intensity Score' is not quantitatively accurate, it served both to regulate the amount of exercise taken and to demonstrate an improvement in physical performance.

This study shows the feasibility and some of the potential beneficial effects of a physical training programme for middle-aged men.

## ACKNOWLEDGEMENTS

This study was carried out with grants from the Sports Council, the Medical Research Council and the British Heart Foundation.

We would like to thank Dr. O. G. Edholm, Head of the M.R.C. Division of Human Physiology, National Institute for Medical Research, London, for his advice and guidance in this study. Assistance in collating the results was provided by Miss Sandra Alder.

The study was based entirely on the system of exercises designed and applied by Mr. Alistair Murray of the City Gymnasium. Without his expert knowledge and enthusiasm, and the practical assistance of Mr. Frank Shipman, also working at the City Gymnasium under a grant from the Sports Council, this work could not have been carried out.

We would also like to thank Dr. Marie Hutchinson and Dr. Steven Spiro of the Royal Postgraduate Medical School and Mr. Tom Reilly of Liverpool Polytechnic for their help with the physiological tests. The biochemical analyses were performed mainly at the Institute of Ophthalmology in Professor Norman Ashton's Department.

TABLE I. Mechanisms by which physical activity may reduce the occurrence or severity of coronary heart disease. (after Fox et al.[11])

*Physical activity may:*

| Increase | Decrease |
| --- | --- |
| *Coronary collateral vascularization* | *Serum levels of:* |
| *Coronary vessel size* | *Cholesterol* |
| *Myocardial efficiency* | *Triglycerides* |
| *Efficiency of peripheral blood distribution and return* | *Free fatty acids* |
| *Fibrinolytic capability* | *Glucose intolerance* |
| *Arterial oxygen content* | *Obesity – adiposity* |
| *Red blood cell mass and blood volume* | *Platelet stickiness* |
| *Thyroid function* | *Arterial blood pressure at rest* |
| *Growth hormone production* | *Heart rate* |
| *Tolerance to stress* | *Vulnerability to dysrhythmias* |
| *Prudent living habits* | *Neurohormonal over-reaction* |
| *'Joie de vivre'* | *Strain associated with psychic 'stress'* |

## REFERENCES

1. *Bannister, R.* British Medical Journal, *1972, 4, 711*
2. *Morris, J. N.* et al. Lancet, *1973, 1, 333*
3. *Carruthers, M.* Lancet, *1973, 1, 1048*
4. *Kilbom, A.* et al. Scandinavian Journal of Clinical Laboratory Investigation, *1969, 24, 315*
5. *Sanne, H. M. and Wilhelmsen, L.* Scandinavian Journal of Rehabilitation Medicine, *1973, 3, 47*
6. *Pyrola, K.* et al. *In* Coronary Heart Disease and Physical Fitness, *ed. Larson, O. A. and Malmborg, R. O. p. 261, Scandinavian University Books, Munksgaard, 1971*
7. *Holloszy, J. O.* et al. American Journal of Cardiology, *1964, 14, 753*
8. *Fitzgerald, O., Heffernan, A. and McFarland, R.* Clinical Science, *1965, 28, 83*
9. *Hoffman, A. A., Nelson, W. R. and Goss, F. A.* American Journal of Cardiology, *1967, 20, 516*
10. *Mann, G. V.* et al. American Journal of Medicine, *1969, 46, 12*
11. *Fox, S. M., Naughton, J. P. and Garman, P. A.* Modern Concepts of Cardiovascular Disease, *1972, Part 1, XLI, 17*

12. *Ewing, D. J.* et al. Lancet, *1975*, 1, *1113*
13. *Borg, G.* Scandinavian Journal of Rehabilitation Medicine, *1970*, 2, *92*
14. *Spiro, S. G.* et al. Clinical Science and Molecular Medicine, *1974*, 46, *191*
15. *Davies, C. T. M.* Clinical Science and Molecular Medicine, *1972*, 42, *1*
16. *Edholm, O. In* Physical Activity in Health and Disease, *ed. Evang, K. and Anderson, K. Scandinavian University Books of Oslo, 1966*
17. *Eysenck, H. J.* The Eysenck Personality Inventory, London: *University of London Press, 1965*
18. *Caine, T. M., Foulds, G. A. and Hope, K.* Manual of the Hostility and Direction of Hostility Questionnaire, London: *London University Press, 1967*
19. *Rahe, R. H.* Proceedings of the Royal Society of Medicine, *1968*, 61, *1124*
20. *Taggart, P. and Carruthers, M.* Lancet, *1972*, 2, *256*
21. *Davies, C. T. M.* et al. European Journal of Applied Physiology, *1974*, 32, *195*
22. *Davies, C. T. M. and Knibbs, A. V.* Internationale Zeitschrift fur Angewandte Physiology, *1971*, 29, *299*
23. *Nordesjö, L. O.* Acta physiologica Scandinavica, *1974, Suppl. 405*
24. *Clausen, J. P., Trap-Jensen, J. and Lassen, N. A.* Scandinavian Journal of Clinical and Laboratory Investigation, *1970*, 26, *295*
25. *Opie, L. H.* Lancet, *1975*, 1, *192*
26. *Raab, W. In* Society, Stress and Disease, *ed. Levi, L. p. 389, London. Oxford University Press, 1971*

## TABLE II. Performance on Cycle Ergometer

| Oxygen uptake ($\dot{V}O_2$) | Mean heart rate ±SD (bts/min) at standard $\dot{V}O_2$ | | Mean ventilation ±SD (l/min). at standard $\dot{V}O_2$ | |
|---|---|---|---|---|
| | 1·0 l/min | 1·5 l/min | 1·0 l/min | 1·5 l/min |
| 1st test | 105·6 ±15·3 | 129·7 ±17·9 | 22·1 ± 3·3 | 37·4 ±3·2 |
| 2nd test (8 weeks later) | 103·0 ±12·0 | 126·0 ±17·9 | 24·7 ±3·4 | 37·0 ±4·4 |
| 3rd test (14 weeks later) | 104·0 ±4·2 | 124·3 ±18·0 | 25·8 ±3·7 | 38·9 ±4·0 |

## TABLE III. Comparison of Activities of all 40 Subjects on Different Days (mean time in minutes/day)

| | Weekday | Saturday | Sunday |
|---|---|---|---|
| Bed | 456 | 474 | 529 |
| Lying | 7 | 20 | 30 |
| Sitting | 628 | 476 | 496 |
| Standing | 82 | 96 | 99 |
| Walking | 101 | 117 | 78 |
| Dressing | 34 | 31 | 27 |
| Driving | 74 | 69 | 46 |
| Gymnasium | 24 | — | — |
| Miscellaneous | 34 | 157 | 134 |

*(The term 'miscellaneous' includes golf, tennis, swimming, sailing, gardening, car-cleaning, household repairs)*

## TABLE IV. Comparison of Weekday Activities of Subjects Working in the City of London and Outside
### *(mean time in minutes/day)*

|               | City (22 men) | Outside City (18 men) |
|---------------|:-------------:|:---------------------:|
| Bed           | 460           | 444                   |
| Lying         | 2             | 18                    |
| Sitting       | 660           | 598                   |
| Standing      | 85            | 85                    |
| Walking       | 104           | 101                   |
| Dressing      | 31            | 38                    |
| Driving       | 59            | 95                    |
| Gymnasium     | 21            | 23                    |
| Miscellaneous | 18            | 38                    |

## TABLE V. The Immediate Effects of Exercise in Healthy Volunteers on Blood Chemistry

| Variable | Time | n | Mean | S.E. | t. | P < |
|---|---|---|---|---|---|---|
| Total Catecholamines ($\mu$g/1) | Pre | 93 | 0·78 | 0·02 | 17·0 | 0·001 |
| | Post | 93 | 1·42 | 0·04 | | |
| Noradrenaline ($\mu$g/1) | Pre | 93 | 0·74 | 0·01 | 14·4 | 0·001 |
| | Post | 93 | 1·20 | 0·03 | | |
| Adrenaline ($\mu$g/1) | Pre | 93 | 0·04 | 0·01 | 11·4 | 0·001 |
| | Post | 93 | 0·22 | 0·02 | | |
| Total Protein (g/100 ml) | Pre | 107 | 7·20 | 0·04 | 11·9 | 0·001 |
| | Post | 107 | 7·52 | 0·04 | | |
| Albumin (g/100 ml) | Pre | 107 | 4·52 | 0·03 | 9·4 | 0·001 |
| | Post | 107 | 4·68 | 0·03 | | |
| Globulin (g/100 ml) | Pre | 107 | 2·66 | 0·03 | 8·1 | 0·001 |
| | Post | 107 | 2·84 | 0·03 | | |
| Free Fatty Acids ($\mu$mol/1) | Pre | 108 | 915 | 35·4 | 0·2 | N.S. |
| | Post | 108 | 918 | 35·9 | | |
| Triglyceride (mg/100 ml) | Pre | 107 | 149 | 8·00 | 0·8 | N.S. |
| | Post | 107 | 148 | 7·86 | | |
| Cholesterol (mg/100 ml) | Pre | 107 | 250 | 3·97 | 5·84 | 0·001 |
| | Post | 107 | 257 | 4·04 | | |
| Glucose (mg/100 ml) | Pre | 104 | 87·6 | 1·75 | 3·53 | 0·001 |
| | Post | 104 | 91·4 | 1·98 | | |
| Lactate (mmol/1) | Pre | 4·2 | 1·7 | 0·12 | 13·0 | 0·001 |
| | Post | 4·2 | 8·6 | 0·52 | | |

# BRITISH PILOT STUDY OF EXERCISE THERAPY

## II. Patients with Cardiovascular Disease

P. Nixon, F.R.C.P.
Consultant Cardiologist,
Charing Cross Hospital,
London, W.6.

M. E. Carruthers, M.D., M.R.C.Path.,
Senior Lecturer,
Department of Chemical Pathology (Research)
St. Mary's Hospital Medical School,
London, W2 1PG

D. J. E. Taylor, M.R.C.P.
H. J. N. Bethell, M.R.C.P.
and
W. Grabau, M.R.C.P.
Formerly Registrars to the Department of
Cardiology, Charing Cross Hospital, London, W.6.

# SUMMARY

Two groups of middle-aged men, one with and one without overt cardiovascular disease, were studied while they were taking part in a specially designed course of exercise therapy in a Gymnasium. The 'patients' group had at least two months pre-treatment to allow physical recovery and mental re-education before their initial very small test dose of exercise. Using short periods of progressive, mainly weight-loaded, isotonic exercises carefully regulated by control of pulse rate and avoidance of symptoms of over-exertion, both groups showed large increases in effort capacity and reductions in resting pulse rate, blood pressure and plasma lipid levels within two months.

The safety of this particular form of exercise was shown in this high-risk population by the low drop-out rate and the absence of cardiovascular accidents in the Gymnasium over a ten year period. It is suggested that, given suitable training of the staff and using the safeguards described, the presence of doctors and a cardiac resuscitation team is unnecessary in a Gymnasium specializing in cardiac rehabilitation. This makes it possible for rehabilitation and physio-therapy departments throughout the country to carry out this effective and positive form of exercise therapy.

# INTRODUCTION

*'The wise for cure on exercise depend'*
*(Dryden, circa 1675)*

The prescription of exercise for various forms of cardiovascular disease is not new, as testified by Heberden's famous reference in 1818 to his patient with angina who was 'nearly cured' by the task of sawing wood for half-an-hour every day. Again, Stokes in 1854[1] suggested that 'The symptoms of debility of the heart are often removable by a regulated course of gymnastics or by pedestrian exercise'. As a treatment for 'soldier's heart' gymnastic activity was successfully introduced during the First World War by Sir James Mackenzie. This was such a novelty that half the cardiological establishment of the day attended the first exercise session, and were impressed by the efficacy of the treatment and absence of fatal side effects.

After a period of nearly 50 years, during which vigorous physical activity was regarded as unsuitable for patients with cardiovascular disease, there was a re-awakening of interest during the nineteen-sixties. This happened simultaneously in many parts of the world, including Germany,[2] Scandinavia,[3,4] America,[5,6] Israel[7] and the UK.[8,9] The regimens used and results obtained have been reviewed by Kellerman,[10] Raab[11] and Sanne.[12] Except for the work of Groden[13] and Carson,[14] there has been a remarkable absence of practical work in cardiac rehabilitation in Britain, although the joint working party on this subject set up by the Royal College of Physicians and British Cardiac Society may help to establish the recommendations of the World Health Organization.[15]

The subjects chosen for this British study were two groups of middle-aged men, one with and one without cardiovascular disease, who were undergoing exercise therapy in a Gymnasium. The purpose of the exercise therapy was to obtain maximum fitness rapidly and *safely. It had been held that this combination of exercise and informal group therapy would appeal to the noradrenaline-addicted coronary-prone individual whose restless, driving predisposition to over-activity could be harnessed to the creation of positive health in place of destruction from fatigue and tension.*[16]

*There are several reasons for choosing this particular Gymnasium for the study. Firstly, the principle of 'do no harm' was a major concern. The Gymnasium chosen offered personal supervision by an experienced remedial gymnast, Alistair Murray, who had already developed a carefully regulated and progressive exercise system for cardiac patients under the responsibility of one of us (P.N.). The system enabled patients to relate their monitored progress to causes of fatigue and anxiety in their daily lives. Secondly, it was a system amenable to study and quantitation in relation to established physiological methods.*[17]

## SUBJECTS AND METHODS

*The subjects studied undertook a course of exercise at the Gymnasium, lasting at least two months. They were divided into two groups, (a) 'Volunteers' – of a total of 1535 middle-aged men attending the Gymnasium, not on medical advice, but because they wished to become fitter, 71 volunteered for this part of the study. Their ages were 35–60 (mean 44·2) years. The consent of their General Practitioner for them to take part in the study was obtained prior to the first examination. Each attended the Cardiac Department at Charing Cross Hospital for history-taking, clinical examination, electrocardiography at rest and after exercise, and for assessment of left ventricular function by phonocardiography and apexcardiography.*[18,19] *Fifty-four (76%) were considered to be normal, 10 (14%) to be hypertensive and 7 (10%) had abnormal left ventricular function without hypertension.*

*At the Gymnasium, 63 of the 'volunteers' had monthly readings of resting pulse rate and blood pressure, measured with a Hawkesley Zero Muddling Sphygmomanometer recorded for up to six months from starting the training programme.*

*(b) 'Patients' (excluding above). These were a total of 248 males, referred by a consultant cardiologist (P.N.), their ages being 22–74 (mean 52) years, of whom 17 (7%) had cardiac neurosis, 18 (7%) were hypertensive (BP 150/90 or above), 74 (29%) had pre-infarction syndrome,*[20,21] *66 (28%) had ischaemic heart disease without infarction and 73 (29%) were post-infarction patients.*

# THE PREPARATIONS FOR GYMNASIUM EXERCISE

'Volunteers' usually had begun exercise before tests started, and with two exceptions, those in whom the tests revealed hypertension or early ischaemic heart disease continued to exercise, but were managed as 'patients'. 'Patients', before they visited the Gymnasium, underwent at least two months pre-treatment. This period was regarded as a most important part of the rehabilitation programme which, as well as allowing time for recovery from infarction and the rich development of the coronary collateral circulation,[22] permitted considerable patient self-examination and education; and taught them techniques for avoiding the overstrained state preceding breakdown in health in general[23] and regarded as preceding coronary illness in particular.[21] This involved control of anger-provoking situations, and where these could not be avoided, the use of diazepam to remain calm during the day and to obtain adequate sleep at night. Apart from thiazide diuretics in a few patients, no further medication was used.

Although walking at gradually increasing pace and for progressively increasing distances was encouraged during this period, patients were trained to avoid both the physical and the emotional triggers of cardiac pain. Practical experience of rehabilitation quickly taught the lesson that great expansion of cardiac performance was possible only where the patient disciplined himself to avoid producing this pain in his daily life, usually by paying attention to time pressures and sources of anger, frustration, resentment or righteous indignation. We agree with the proposition that conflicts at work and in the family, changes in working conditions, life events of especial importance and absence from work through illness, namely the conditions that predispose to high levels of catecholamine secretion, are especially related to the onset of myocardial infarction and sudden death.[24]

Patients were required not to use β-blockers or coronary vasodilators, e.g. trinitrin. They were not nagged to stop smoking or to lose weight until they had recovered from the overstrained state and were actively engaged at the Gymnasium. Once there, control could usually be achieved by maintaining a constant calorie intake in the presence of increased energy expenditure. The desires to eat and drink excessively and to smoke subsided as fitness waxed and strain waned.

Towards the end of the pre-treatment period, the patient visited the Gymnasium with his wife or another relation. This provided an overall impression of the Gymnasium and the chance to discuss any anxieties with the Gymnasium staff: the visit allayed fears that the

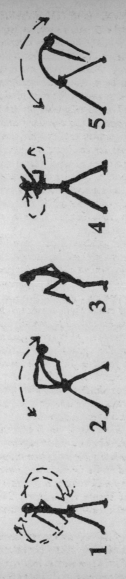

*Gymnasium activity might be uncomfortable or too strenuous.*

When the patients began to attend the City Gymnasium regularly, they were exposed to three influences: Firstly, lessons from the medical and Gymnasium staff about the effects of emotional stress and fatigue on cardiac performance. Secondly, informal 'group therapy' where new patients and older members could communicate with one another over a cup of caffeine-free coffee in the Gymnasium. Thirdly, the influence of the exercise itself.

## INITIAL EXERCISE SESSION

After the 'volunteers' and 'patients' had changed into gym kit, the pulse rate was taken. If this 'arrival' pulse rate was over 90 beats per minute, the subject was asked to sit and rest until it had fallen below this level. Then the test dose of five light, mobilizing exercises illustrated in fig. 1 were carried out to ease all the major muscles and joints over their full range of movement. Each exercise was performed 12 times, and the test dose ended with one minute on a lightly loaded cycle ergometer. The subject was closely watched throughout for the onset of discomfort, distress or pallor, which would be taken as a signal to stop the test. It was undesirable for the pulse rate to be more than 110 at the end of these exercises. The response to the test dose enabled the therapist to choose an exercise programme which fitted the patient's age and observed condition, or revealed that he was not ready for exercise therapy.

## EXERCISE PROGRAMME

All exercise sessions began with the mobilizing exercises of the test dose, taking less than five minutes, and continued with the 10 separate exercises described and characterized in physiological and biochemical terms in the previous paper.[17] The system used was the 'Murray Method of Progressive Exercise by Pulse Control' with measurable work intensity. All subjects started with very low work intensities using weights of only 2–3 lbs. They were taught to count their pulse rate by palpation at the wrist, but during the exercise programme it was quicker and more convenient to use an ECG-heart-rate meter* activated by grasping two electrodes.

By means of this schedule of 10 different exercises graded in 'Repounds per minute', the subject's pulse rate was kept within the 'pulse range' appropriate to his age and condition, as indicated in fig. 2, for the 10 to 15 minutes of the active exercise period. Exercising week by week, without exceeding the prescribed heart rate, and
* Murray Pulse Monitor M.I.E. Ltd.

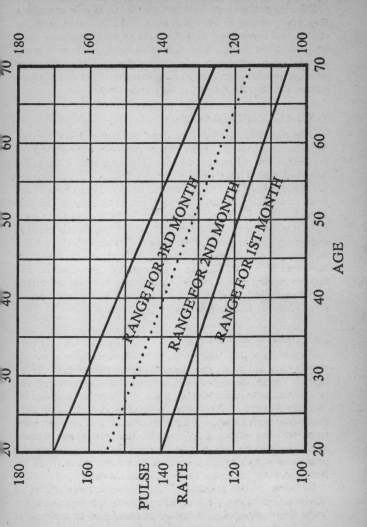

*without creating sensations of more than moderate effort, the subject was able to accomplish this programme with slower pulse rates and greater ease. As his physical condition improved the intensity of the work was increased by raising the rate of movement, the number of repetitions, and reducing the rest pauses between exercises. When the rest pauses had been eliminated, and the number of repetitions raised to a maximum of 20 to 30 for each large muscle group exercise, the subjects were allowed to increase the weights used by a small amount. Whenever the weight was increased, the rate of movement and number of repetitions were reduced, the rest pauses reintroduced, and the progression was repeated.*

*Subjects recorded the intensity of their exercise in 'Repounds' per minute at weekly intervals. Usually a plateau of fitness was reached by patients after two to three months. Important advantages of this self-assessment of exercise intensity was the measurable progress in the first two to three months of exercise, and the ability of the subject to demonstrate to his own satisfaction that a morbid life-style, produced for example by over-work, anger, frustration, could predictably reduce his capacity for physical exertion.*

*Although isometric work is avoided, exercises which are largely isotonic are also unsuitable for cardiac patients when the resistance to be overcome is so great that the movement can be repeated only a few times. Examples include an overweight person attempting full knee bends, 'sit-ups' from a horizontal position, or press-ups from the floor. Similarly, even away from the Gymnasium, patients were warned against such mainly isometric exertions as pushing a car, pulling on the wheel of a heavy car when parking, undoing stiff bolts or screws or, as was reported to have brought on one of Churchill's heart attacks, straining at a jammed window.*

*Thirty of the normal 'volunteers', and all the patients with cardiovascular disease, returned to the Cardiology Department of Charing Cross Hospital for repetition of the full range of cardiological tests. Serial lipid estimations were carried out weekly on 12 of the patients with coronary heart disease, cholesterol and triglyceride being measured by the standard AA11-24 method, and free fatty acids by a fluorescence method.[25]*

## RESULTS

*The drop-out rate during the first two months in both 'volunteers' and 'patients' was low (5%). The reasons given for discontinuing included transport problems in attending the Gymnasium, and temporary exacerbation of pre-existing musculo-skeletal disabilities.*

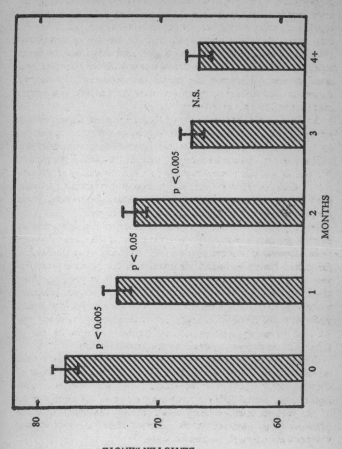

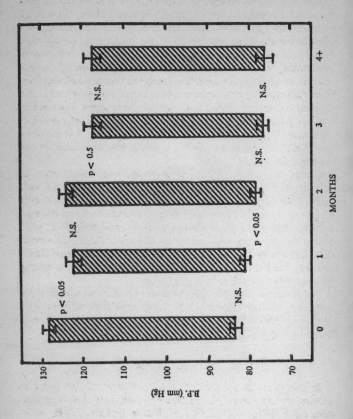

*In approximately 500 'patients' there were no cases of cardiac arrest, infarction or collapse in the Gymnasium and none suffered any form of cardiac emergency. This also applies to the total of over 2,000 other members attending the Gymnasium during the past 10 years. Of the 248 patients with cardiovascular disease studied, nine died during the three year period of the study, none during their initial two month term of rehabilitation. Of these, one died of pneumonia, one of sub-acute bacterial endocarditis, one of carcinomatosis, one, aged 74, of a cerebrovascular accident, one of congestive heart failure, and two of unknown causes some months or years after finishing a course of rehabilitation at the Gymnasium. The remaining two patients suffered sudden cardiac arrest during periods of emotional disturbance: in one, the arrest occurred while watching the World Cup match on television, and in the other while he was visiting his mother in hospital.*

*Of the 30 normal 'volunteers' who were re-examined after an average of a year's exercise, no significant change in the more detailed cardiological indices were found. However, there were progressive reductions in resting pulse rates and blood pressure with training (figs. 3 and 4). In the 248 'patients', gallop rhythms faded, blood pressures approached normality and minor E.C.G. abnormalities often resolved during the pre-treatment phase. In no case did the course of exercise result in any deterioration in the objective tests of left ventricular function.*

*The reduction in plasma lipid levels during a two months period of exercise in 12 patients with I.H.D., together with the increase in the intensity of the exercise which they were able to perform, is shown in fig. 5.*

## DISCUSSION

*In this study, exercise was found to be very safe, probably on account of the emphasis given to the 'pre-treatment' and the precautions taken during the build-up in physical activity. It also maintained the improvement in cardiac condition which had begun during the pre-treatment phase. This was in contrast to other similar but undisciplined and non-exercising patients of the Cardiac Department, who appeared to have higher relapse rates as measured by re-admission, persistent or recurrent pain, deterioration of left ventricular function, or the need either to continue or augment hypotensive regimes. The increase in effort capacity of these patients treated by exercise therapy was clinically far more impressive than that obtained by either β-blockade or surgery.*

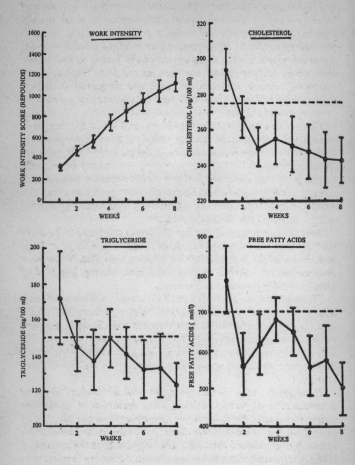

Some 'patients' did relapse, usually a year or so after ceasing exercise, and responded well to a further course of rest, pre-treatment and Gymnasium attendance. The decreases in resting pulse rate and blood pressure in the 'volunteers' were similar to those usually reported with other physical training programmes using dynamic (isotonic) exercises.[26] An important feature of the schedules carried out in this Gymnasium is that they were light 'weight loaded' rather than severe 'weight lifting' exercises, as the latter involve static (isometric) muscle contractions which are dangerous in hypertensive subjects[27] and those who may be approaching cerebral or coronary vascular illness.

There is considerable variability in the evidence on the changes in plasma lipids which occur during prolonged exercise programmes. Reductions in cholesterol reported in some studies[28,29,30] were not found in others.[6,31,32] These conflicting results may be partially explained by the work of Taylor[33] which indicated that exercise reduced serum cholesterol most markedly when people on a high fat intake lost weight or when only the carbohydrate content of the diet was increased to keep the weight constant.

Similarly, reports of lowering of plasma triglyceride by exercise[30,31] were not confirmed by Mann et al.[34] whose subjects, however, increased the amount of carbohydrate in their diet. No previous observations on changes in free fatty acids during a period of exercise could be found in the literature.

The results of this study indicated that, given a constant dietary intake with regard to carbohydrate and fat, significant and clinically potentially useful reductions in all three of the lipid fractions measured were obtained using this exercise regime (fig. 5). The decreases began within three months and were maintained, except during gross emotional upheavals, for as long as the exercise was continued.

These effects on the plasma lipids were probably brought about by a combination of factors. Although the reduction in total body weight was small, averaging 0·5–1 kg per month in the majority of cases, there was a considerable decrease in body fat as measured by estimations of skinfold thickness. This suggests that the amount of metabolically active muscle in the body was increasing in relation to body fat. This would explain previous reports that the fit can oxidise fatty acids more effectively than the unfit,[35] and even at rest mobilize and utilize more fat.[36]

The consequent reduction in the amount of free fatty acid available for triglyceride and cholesterol synthesis can also account for the lowering of both these lipid fractions, and the failure of triglyceride levels[36] and cholesterol levels[37] to increase with age in groups maintaining a high level of physical activity, and hence remaining lean and muscular.

In addition to the somatic effects of exercise therapy, attendance at the Gymnasium appeared to provide psychological benefit. Apart from health education provided by the Gymnasium staff, the patients were encouraged to discuss their problems and successes among themselves in informal group therapy. In reply to a questionnaire given to men who had completed two months' exercise, the majority reported that they felt they were coping better with problems at work and at home, were less tired at the end of the day, and slept better at night, in addition to having a greater capacity for physical work. Similar mood changes in response to a course of exercise in cardiac patients are commonly noted[5,6] and, by reducing catecholamine secretion rates, may contribute to the lowering of plasma lipids.

During this study of carefully supervised Gymnasium activity, several principles have emerged which we believe are of importance in the prescription of exercise therapy for unfit individuals and those with cardiovascular disease. Above all, there is the need for safety precautions in any course of exercises for unfit adults or patients with cardiovascular disease, particularly in the early stages. This need is underlined by the presence of unsuspected abnormalities in nearly a quarter of the group of self-selected 'volunteers'. The precautions include an initial cardiological examination, adequate pre-treatment, provision of suitable conditions for exercise, skilled supervision, individual self-regulation of the intensity of the exercise at each stage, the avoidance of anything approaching maximal or isometric exercise, and the prevention of competition with other Gymnasium members.[38]

Pre-treatment as a literally vital preliminary to a course of vigorous exercise for patients with cardiovascular disease has been described earlier in this article. 'Volunteers' more than 20% over their ideal weight are generally advised to get within this limit before vigorous exercise is undertaken. The more unfit and elderly people should also gradually prepare themselves over a period of about two months by graduated walking, going on to stair climbing or stepping on and off a box a foot high for periods increasing to several minutes each day.

If the subjects are to relax and enjoy the exercise, the conditions under which it is carried out must be comfortable. In particular, cold must be avoided because it has a marked pressor effect in many individuals, increasing the likelihood of muscle stiffness, and is conducive to angina. Timing of the exercise session is also important, as most people derive more benefit from exercise in the mid-morning or before lunch, rather than at the end of a heavy day at work.

By convention, the duration of an exercise session is usually three-quarters of an hour or more. This study, and those of Sanne[12] and Nordesjö,[39] suggest that given a suitable work intensity, the period can be shortened to between 15 and 30 minutes without loss of training effect, providing the frequency is three times per week. Such a reduction lessens the demands on the subject's time and motivation, lowering drop-out rates. It also means that the three shortened exercise sessions each week pioneered 10 years ago by Alistair Murray, and regarded as optimal in the later Scandinavian studies, can be fitted comfortably into a normal lunch-hour break, and still leave time for a shower, changing and light refreshments. The creation of pleasant conditions is of great importance in making exercise sufficiently addictive to become a lifelong habit. Just as the majority of benefits in terms of increased physical fitness and reduced lipid levels appear within two or three months of starting exercise, so they disappear within two or three months of stopping. Spartan gymnasium conditions and group exercises may revive unpleasant memories of compulsory physical training at school or in the Army. Similarly, attending a hospital gymnasium[14] may be unacceptable to some of the anxiety-driven patients who may be most at risk from recurrence of coronary illness.

The system of gymnasium exercise taught the patient to vary the intensity of his exercise, within the prescribed margins, according to fluctuations in his general condition, by heightening his awareness of fatigue and dyspnoea, and teaching him to make use of his pulse rate. The lessons did not increase anxiety and introspection, but provided a biofeedback and control system that increased confidence and satisfied the patient's need to play an active part in the regulation of his recovery. They were most useful in helping the patient to understand the effects of changes in life-style upon his physical condition.

Instead of stopping increasingly frequently to check pulse rates, as the course continued the subjects generally begin to rely more on their subjective sensations, with only occasional measurements to confirm that they were staying within the prescribed pulse rate zone. We suggest that other forms of exercise for unfit middle-aged people, such as cycling, swimming and jogging could also be made safe by training people to regulate the intensity of exertion according to subjective sensations and pulse rates.

Competition between members is discouraged, as it results in noradrenaline secretion and its undesirable circulatory and metabolic side effects,[40] and may also lead to over-exertion.[38] This point is also emphasized by Sanne,[12] but is not a feature of the regime described by Gottheiner,[7] whose article showed four of his fitter post-infarction patients competing in a 60 metre sprint race, or Kavanagh et al.[41] whose patients took part in marathon races. Group work is undesirable in comparison to individual supervision because it must encourage over-activity in some and under-activity in others.

If supervision is not provided the patient's own choice of exercise after myocardial infarction is usually inappropriate in intensity, frequency, duration and type. Some remain as invalids unnecessarily. Others endanger themselves by adopting a 'paradoxical and blatantly illogical' denial of obvious disability[42,43] and attempting unrealistic achievements.

Intensive courses of cardiac rehabilitation in residential centres are offered by the Royal Air Force to Servicemen, but are not yet generally available within the N.H.S. They may be of special value where the main causes of the breakdown in health are in the home.

The absence of cardiovascular accidents in this series suggests that the presence of doctors and a cardiac resuscitation team is unnecessary in a Gymnasium specializing in cardiac rehabilitation if the safeguards described are followed. It should be possible for patients with cardiovascular disease to obtain a three month course with three sessions each week at a specially organized 'school' within the Physiotherapy Department of their district hospital, and then 'graduate' to join their non-medical friends in a Gymnasium run by the local health authority or privately, providing they have been specially trained in this type of work and that strict adherence to these principles of safe exercise continues.[44] A trial of introducing this system of training in the Physiotherapy Department of an N.H.S. hospital is currently in progress. Another novel feature of this type of exercise is that it would enable some patients to continue 'extramural' studies at home, encouraged by audiovisual aids such as records and tapes, together with brief refresher courses at the hospital training school.

## ACKNOWLEDGEMENTS

This work was carried out with grants from the Sports Council, the Medical Research Council and the British Heart Foundation. The late Dr. Harold Lewis of the M.R.C. initiated this study of cardiac rehabilitation.

We would like to thank Dr. O. G. Edholm, Head of the M.R.C.

Division of Human Physiology, National Institute for Medical Research, London, for his advice and guidance.

The study was based entirely on the system of exercises designed and applied by Mr. Alistair Murray of the City Gymnasium. Without his expert knowledge and enthusiasm, and the practical assistance of Mr. Frank Shipman, also working in the City Gymnasium under a grant from the Sports Council, this work could not have been carried out. The biochemical analyses were performed mainly at the Institute of Ophthalmology, and we would like to thank the Medical Research Council for an equipment grant, and Professor Norman Ashton for laboratory facilities. Able technical help was provided by Miss Eileen Willmott.

## REFERENCES

1. Stokes, W. In Diseases of the Heart and Aorta, London, 1854
2. Beckman, P. In Prevention of Ischaemic Heart Disease, ed. Raab, W. p. 393, Springfield, Illinois, 1966
3. Saltin, B. et al. Circulation, 1968, Suppl. 7
4. Clausen, J. P., Larson, O. A. and Trap-Jensen, J. Circulation, 1969, 40, 143
5. Hellerstein, H. K. and Hornstein, T. R. Journal of Rehabilitation, 1966, 32, 38
6. Naughton, J., Bruhn, J. and Lategola, M. I. American Journal of Medicine, 1969, 46, 725
7. Gottheiner, V. American Journal of Cardiology, 1968, 22, 426
8. Nixon, P. and Murray, A. Heart, 1969, September issue, p. 5
9. Nixon, P. Health Visitor, 1970, 43, 356
10. Kellerman, J. J. Acta Cardiologica, 1970, Suppl. 14, p. 61
11. Raab, W. In Society, Stress and Disease, ed. Levi, L. p. 389, Oxford University Press, London, 1971
12. Sanne, H. Acta Medica Scandinavica, 1973, Suppl. 551
13. Groden, B. M., Semple, T. and Shaw, G. B. British Heart Journal, 1971, 33, 756
14. Carson, P. et al. British Medical Journal, 1974, 3, 213
15. World Health Organization. Report of Regional Office for Europe, Copenhagen, 1969
16. Nixon, P. Rehabilitation, 1972, 81, 23
17. Carruthers, M. Nixon P. Murray M. Lancet 1975, 1, 447
18. Taylor, D. J. and Nixon, P. British Heart Journal, 1972, 34, 905

19. *Nixon, P. In* Angina Pectoris, *ed. Oglesby, P. MedCom Press, New York, 1974*

20. *Nixon, P.* Practitioner, *1973*, 211, *5*

21. *Nixon, P. and Bethell, H. J. N.* American Journal of Cardiology, *1974*, 33, *446*

22. *Blumgart, H. L.* et al. Circulation, *1950*, 1, *10*

23. *Kennedy, A.* Lancet, *1957*, 1, *261*

24. *Theorell, T.* et al. Psychosomatic Medicine, *1972*, 34, *505*

25. *Carruthers, M. and Young, D. A. B.* Clinica Chimica Acta, *1973*, 49, *341*

26. *Yarvote, P. M.* et. al. Journal of Occupational Medicine, *1974*, 16, *589*

27. *Ewing, D. J.* et al. British Heart Journal, *1973*, 35, *413*

28. *Naughton, J. and Blake, B.* American Journal of Medical Science, *1964*, 247, *286*

29. *Fitzgerald, O., Hefferman, A. and McFarland, R.* Clinical Science, *1965*, 28, *83*

30 *Hoffman, A. A., Nelson, W. R. and Goss, F. A.* American Journal of Cardiology, *1967*, 20, *516*

31. *Holloszy, J. O.* et al. American Journal of Cardiology, *1964*, 14, *753*

32. *Durbeck, D. C., Heinzelmann, F. and Schacter, J.* American Journal of Cardiology, *1972*, 30, *784*

33. *Taylor, H. L. In* Work and the Heart, *ed. Rosenbaum, F. F. and Belknap, E. L. P. B. Hoeber, New York, 1959*

34. *Mann, G. V.* et al. American Journal of Medicine, *1969*, 46, *12*

35. *Johnson, R. H.* et al. Lancet, *1969*, 2, *452*

36. *Hurter, F. R.* et al. Lancet, *1972*, 2, *671*

37. *Ho, K. J.* et al. Archives of Pathology, *1971*, 91, *387*

38. *Opie, L. H.* Lancet, *1975*, 1, *263*

39. *Nordesjö, L.* Acta physiologica Scandinavica, *1974, Suppl. 405*

40. *Carruthers, M. and Taggart, P.* American Heart Journal, *1974*, 88, *1*

41. *Kavanagh, T., Shephard, R. H. and Pondit, V.* Journal of the American Medical Association, *1974*, 229, *1602*

42. *Chambers, W. N. and Reiser, M. F.* Psychosomatic Medicine, *1953*, 15, *38*

43. *Hackett, T. P. and Cassen, N. H.* American Journal of Cardiology, *1969*, 24, *651*

44. *Carruthers, M. and Murray, A.* F/40 *Futura Publications Ltd, London*